YOUR FUTURE IS IN YOUR HANDS

YOUR FUTURE IS IN YOUR HANDS

22 KEYS TO CREATING A LIFE YOU LOVE BEFORE IT'S TOO LATE

LORETTA LUBERA

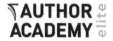

Published by Author Academy Elite
PO Box 43, Powell, OH 43065
www.AuthorAcademyElite.com

Identifiers:
Library of Congress Control Number: 2021918573
ISBN: 978-1-64746-898-9 (paperback)
ISBN: 978-1-64746-899-6 (hardback)
ISBN: 978-1-64746-900-9 (ebook)

Available in paperback, hardback, e-book, and audiobook.

All scripture quotations, unless otherwise indicated, are taken from the Holy Bible, New Living Translation, copyright 1996, 2004, 2007, 2015 by Tyndale House Foundation. Used by permission of Tyndale House Publishers, Inc., Carol Stream, Illinois 60188. All rights reserved worldwide.

Any Internet addresses (websites, blogs, etc.) and telephone numbers printed in this book are offered as a resource. They are not intended in any way to be or imply an endorsement by Author Academy Elite, nor does Author Academy Elite vouch for the content of these sites and numbers for the life of this book.

Names and identifying characteristics were disguised to protect the privacy of the individuals who have shared their stories; some details were added or altered for narrative purposes.

Illustrations by Pottery Chan
Portraits in Chapter 4 by Elsa Tsang
Author Photograph by Kevin Lubera
Interior and Cover Design by Jetlaunch

This book is dedicated to my parents,
from whom I have learned more than a lifetime's
worth of invaluable lessons.
I am grateful for their unconditional encouragement,
boundless inspiration, and immeasurable sacrifices.

TABLE OF CONTENTS

INTRODUCTION 1

1 YOU'RE STRONGER THAN YOU THINK 5

2 BE GROUNDED IN JOY 13

3 STAY TRUE TO YOURSELF 23

4 MAKE TIME FOR YOUR PASSION 37

5 YOUR WORDS ARE POWERFUL 55

6 RESTRAIN YOUR PRIDE 65

7 SET GOALS. 73

8 PAUSE TO REFLECT 87

9 MAXIMIZE YOUR SCHOOL YEARS 97

10 SELF-DISCIPLINE IS A GIFT 107

11 MASTER YOUR FINANCES 121

12 ENRICH YOUR SOCIAL NETWORK 135

13 MENTORS ARE ANGELS IN DISGUISE. 145

14 IT'S OKAY TO FAIL 155

15 LEARN TO LOVE TO LEARN. 167

16 BE KIND, UNCONDITIONALLY. 179

17 FIRST, BE THE RIGHT ONE 189

18 KNOW WHAT YOU WANT IN A SPOUSE 201

19 PARENTS ARE HUMAN TOO 221

20 SAY I LOVE YOU OFTEN 231

21 EACH AGE LASTS ONLY ONE YEAR 241

22 YOU ARE WONDERFULLY MADE 257

ACKNOWLEDGMENTS 260

INTRODUCTION

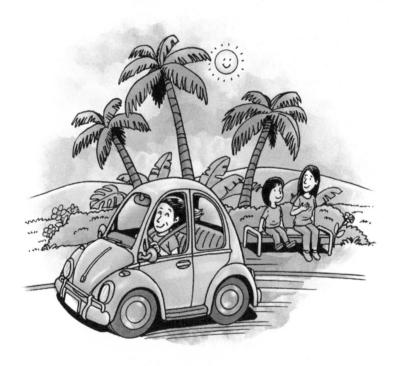

Have you ever experienced moments where inspiration—an idea—pops into your head and refuses to leave?

Two years ago, as I was driving one beautiful morning in Hawai'i, a thought came to mind.

What if you were to write a book on a variety of life lessons to help our younger generation, to impart wisdom so they can learn from the failures and successes of others, and to get ahead in life? Now, these wouldn't be merely your insights, but they'd come from a range of people—perhaps people from around the world—so there are more people from all walks of life to learn from.

Nice idea, I thought.

I went on driving and tucked that thought away.

Days went by, and that idea would not leave me alone. It refused to stay quiet and nudged me again and again.

Soon, I realized this was a calling for me. I had a big purpose, a new assignment—to get this book together and share it with the world.

With that realization came the follow-through. Deep inside, I knew if I were to be able to help someone—even if only one individual—all the efforts behind this book would be worth it.

It's important to learn from our own mistakes. However, if we have the opportunity to avoid heartaches by learning from *others'* mistakes, isn't that even better? And if we can understand what helped set others up for success, wouldn't we want to know more about it?

If there is a way for us to get to a meaningful life—one we actually *love*—by applying other people's experiences and learnings, why would we say no?

When we are young, we tend to think we have all the answers. However, there is one thing we lack and cannot replace—experience. And experience comes with time. So, those further along in life who have gained experiences offer us a priceless gift to learn through the lenses of their lives.

A better me, a better you, simply by studying others' life lessons and applying them to our lives.

At first, I didn't quite know how to get started. I mentioned this concept to several people and received contagious enthusiasm. I started to float the question: "What would you tell your younger self if you had a chance?" What I quickly noticed was typically, at least one thing rolled right off their tongue, as though it had been sitting in a corner of their heart, waiting for an opportunity to release. Most of these had a remorseful tone to it, the "I wish I had . . ." and "I wish I hadn't . . ." and the weight of their regrets saddened me. But we are imperfect beings, living imperfect lives. Regrets are often a part of the deal.

I reached out to friends, family, and acquaintances to ask them to share their stories and experiences. From there, I asked them to share the same question with their networks all over the world, to contribute to this project. I am grateful for all the wisdom, honest truths, and vulnerability generously given to make this book a reality. One thing that stood out was love. Behind all the faces, voices, and spoken words, love shone the most. It was as though these people were actually standing in front of their younger selves, taking advantage of ten minutes to leave behind words of wisdom, words of *love*. They wanted their younger selves to do well in life, perhaps because they already knew how their future would turn out or wanted something better for their younger selves.

Life is full of choices. And this book sheds light on the consequences of choices other people have made. Some made choices they were proud of, others not so much. These people faced decisions that you may come across in your life. They understand what you are going through and will likely go through. I hope this book, through its multiple lenses, can guide you to make better decisions because *YOUR FUTURE IS IN YOUR HANDS*. You have the power to shape your future through the choices you make and to create a life you love.

So, here we are. A curation of life stories—good and bad—to help you look at your life and future with a different perspective. You can read the chapters in any order you wish. If certain chapters don't seem relevant to your current life stage, I would encourage you to read them now anyway so you can start planting seeds for the future. Then, you can revisit at a later time with fresh eyes and likely a different way to leverage the lessons. At the end of each chapter, you'll find key takeaways. They might come in handy on days when you need a bit of a reminder or uplifting.

Hopefully, this book will guide you to fewer regrets, greater joy, and a more fulfilling and purposeful future. Thank you for allowing me to be a part of your journey.

Learn from the mistakes of others. You can't live long enough to make them all yourself.

—Eleanor Roosevelt

1

YOU'RE STRONGER
THAN YOU THINK

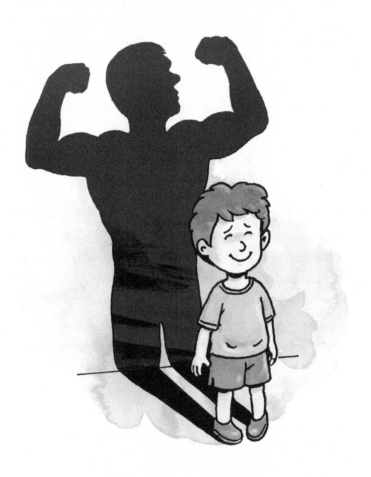

Strength doesn't come from what you can do. It comes from overcoming the things you once thought you couldn't.

—Rikki Rogers

Life can get tough sometimes. There will be days when you will want to throw in the towel. I hope those days don't outnumber the good days. But I also sincerely hope you do have some not-so-great days because it's the peaks and valleys that make life exciting and worth living. Sure, a relatively uneventful life is fine; it's safe. It's like driving on a very long, straight road. The scenery may be nice, but the ride can get dull over time. Soon, you might catch yourself on cruise control mode, just coasting and barely even noticing the beautiful scenery.

Similarly, the blah days make us appreciate the good days more.

Victories are sweeter when you've poured in your blood and sweat.

The dark valleys make being able to stand on the top of the mountain so much more worth celebrating. The dark valleys prove to us that we are stronger than we think.

CELEBRATE YOUR WINS

Success is not relative. If you're elated with an A on an assignment, you should be just as elated when your friend gets an A+. Don't rank yourself against others' achievements. Recognize your growth and the payoff of your hard work. Just because someone does well doesn't mean you *aren't* doing well.

We often fall into this mindset. It's detrimental yet natural to compare ourselves against others. Somehow, our achievements carry less weight when someone else seems to be even more successful. Even within a group of friends who support each other, there is often a psychological stack-ranking. I know a circle of friends who laugh and cry together. But when it comes to talking about their jobs and career paths, one friend shrinks to a state of inferiority, feeling less worthy because of her lack of career achievements. They all genuinely love her just the same. Sure, her job title isn't as fancy as some other ones, but so what? They love her just the same.

Let's not discredit your achievements. Celebrate your wins, no matter how small they may seem. You can do amazing things in life. Don't hold yourself back. Consider a failure or a mistake as a necessary step to get you to where you need to be. Remember, you've had quite a lot of practice *failing*, like a baby learning to walk, like a child learning to ride a bike, as a student trying to ace every assignment and test, as a young person trying to get a job. Keep in mind that *no one is waiting for you to fail.* You are likely the only one bracing for your failure. But if you prepare for the possibility to fail, failure will lose its sting. Embrace the fact that your learning process may not be flawless or graceful. You may continue to take minute baby steps; you may even stumble backward. But when you finally get to your goal, you will look back and celebrate because you will have proved it's all possible.

A STRONG WILL CAN MOVE MOUNTAINS
JOANNE'S STORY

I was only in my fifties when my husband passed away. His decline happened so rapidly that suddenly, I found myself having no choice but to take over his company with little guidance. His operations were vast, with multiple divisions and multiple entities. The company's survival and success, along with the livelihood of all the employees, depended on me. So, feeling blindfolded, I dove in with a lot to handle, especially for someone with practically zero knowledge in this industry.

Though I didn't have the memory or energy of a twenty-year-old, I became a student again. What I did have was tenacity and drive. I couldn't let my husband's legacy succumb, not on my watch!

It would have been easier if the business was flourishing when it dropped in my lap. However, as my husband became ill toward the end of his life, the company suffered with him. By the time I took the reins, the threads were increasingly visible. Things were barely holding together, and clients started to notice.

The responsibility tore me in so many different directions. Everything was a priority. It was hard to be doing and learning and managing and fixing all at the same time. The learning curve was the toughest I had ever encountered. I dedicated every extra minute I had to learn, to catch up. And there were really no *extra* minutes. I traveled frequently to attend all sorts of trade shows, workshops, and conventions, to arm myself with industry knowledge in order to relate to our clients, vendors, and employees.

My younger self would have panicked if I were to tell her that in her mid-life, when everyone starts to think about taking things easier and enjoying life, suddenly she would have to take on a multi-million-dollar company in a male-dominant industry. She would probably brush off the mere thought. Perhaps she'd laugh at the prospect of someone entrusting her with such a mammoth responsibility. I would tell her that her determination and refusal to give up would ultimately carry her through. She had a God who could help her do the impossible and would provide her with divine wisdom to guide her. I would assure her that, because of her focus on the end goal and her outright unwillingness to quit, she would not only turn the company around and make it profitable again, but she'd gain respect from a lot of people. She would make her husband proud.

It was a bittersweet moment when the business was ultimately sold. Each asset, equipment, and building ceased to be mine. Despite all the sweat and tears I had invested into this company, it suddenly felt surreal, like it had all been a dream. I had learned so much and gained so much from this experience. In the process, I proved to myself that I was capable of jumping into this enormous challenge with both feet, could maneuver it into a better shape than when I inherited it, and despite not having the confidence at first, I was indeed stronger than I had thought I could ever be.

Anyone can give up; it's the easiest thing in the world to do. But to hold it together when everyone else would understand if you fell apart, that's true strength.

—Unknown

GROWING UP IN THE EXPRESS LANE
JEFFREY'S STORY

I was the oldest of ten children growing up on a farm. During one of my mother's pregnancies, she suffered a fall and almost had a miscarriage. As a result, the doctor prescribed bedrest until the baby came. So, as the two oldest children, my sister and I had to rise up and assume parental roles. We took care of our younger siblings and worked around the house and on the farm. Everywhere we went, my sister and I had to take care of two of our siblings. This forced us to grow up fast.

It wasn't always enjoyable. What kid would want to give up having fun with friends and supervise their younger brothers and sisters all the time? I often resented the heavy burden placed upon me and felt cornered, like I was never given a choice.

As I got older, I appreciated the experience of caring for others at such a young age. It shaped me to naturally seek ways to help others and to serve without expecting anything in return. It was second nature to me to care about making a difference. This proved to be advantageous for my career path. People knew they could count on me. My managers recognized I voluntarily strove to go above and beyond. I may have missed out on part of my childhood, but that served me in the latter part of my life.

WHEN LIFE GIVES YOU LEMONS
BARBARA'S STORY

When I turned forty, my husband got into an accident and could no longer work. It was devastating. We were a dual-income family by need, not by choice. Our expenses alone were more than what my income could cover.

People say when life gives you lemons, make lemonade. Well, let me tell you, we were at a loss for the next steps when one income suddenly vanished. How do you make lemonade out of that?

After a short period of overcoming the shock, anger, and grief, we evaluated options. We found side hustles that could yield cash flow close to what my husband had been earning. It meant we had to make some adjustments to our spending (which was already minimal). We learned that when adversity hits, it's normal to throw your hands up and say, "I can't do this!" But when you have children depend on you to figure it out and watch how you respond to challenges, you find a strength you didn't know you had and push through. Somehow, one way or another, you discover a path. You realize you have more grit than you ever thought.

Always remember you are braver than you believe, stronger than you seem, smarter than you think, and loved more than you know.

—Winnie the Pooh by A. A. Milne

TAKEAWAYS

- You may realize how much stronger you are than you think when quitting isn't an option. When you encounter a problem, remove giving up as an option and find ways to push through. There is always a way.

- Celebrate your wins, big or small. Don't discredit a win simply because it appears dwarfed against someone else's. Let your win be your win.

- We may not always understand our trials, but trust there is a purpose. One day it will make sense.

2

BE GROUNDED IN JOY

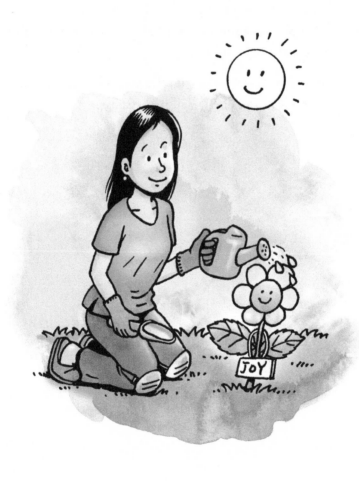

The key to being happy is knowing you have the power to choose what to accept and what to let go.

—Dodinsky

Ultimately, you are in control of your happiness. But when you cannot control the situation or people around you, learn to let it go. Yes, it's easier said than done, and it will take some time, but it will be good for your soul to stop agonizing over things you can't control and can't change.

It took me a while to understand the difference between happiness and joy. Happiness is more circumstantial; it often depends on what's happening in the moment, centered around life's circumstances. Joy, however, is more inherent. One can be joyful even when things aren't going well. Joy has underlying, sustained contentment. It makes you smile and brings you peace even if you may no longer have a reason to smile.

Joy allows you to respond to life's adversities with a positive outlook. It helps you to find the brighter side.

Joy has hope.

A lot of times it boils down to your mindset. Do you find yourself blaming your circumstances, external factors, or other people? Do you catch yourself often in a *grass is greener on the other side* mentality? Do you envy what others have and feel bitter that you lack these possessions?

Being appreciative of what you do have can make a world of difference. Dwelling on the negatives may suck you into a downward spiral and further into a deep, dark place of resentment, which is tough to climb out of. Instead, look at what you do have going well for you. Count your blessings—not your misfortunes—and practice gratitude for every good in your life. If that seems like a daunting task, perhaps it's because there is indeed a lot of good.

Choose to be joyful. When you catch yourself thinking a negative thought, consciously stop it in its tracks and pivot. Outright refuse to fester in negativity and actively direct your thoughts to something more positive. Commit to stop feeling sorry for yourself, stop laying blame, stop finger-pointing. You have control over your happiness, your outlook, your attitude. If you think you have nothing going for you, then you're probably simply not seeing it, and it isn't that no good exists in your life. Perhaps your perspective needs to change.

Someone once said to me, "Is it a problem, or is it merely an inconvenience?" That one simple question stuck with me for years and continues to serve me as an assessment tool in both personal and work settings. We encounter a lot of obstacles in life. If we pause and think about it, we may realize a lot of what we consider problems are actually only inconveniences. These things may cause us to take a bit of a detour or demand a little more time to arrive at the end goal. But it's not truly a *problem*. We may perceive it as a problem because we're frustrated having to go out of our way, which disrupts our plans, stalls our progress, and we feel like we are no longer in control. However, when we realize it's simply an inconvenience, we can take a deep breath and tackle it with a calmer demeanor. There is light at the end of the tunnel—though the tunnel may be a little longer than we had expected—we only need to keep pushing forward.

BEAUTY THAT COUNTS
LAURA'S STORY

Growing up, I had my fair share of insecurity over my body and my complexion. It certainly didn't help that my acne wouldn't leave me alone for good. And my body inflated and deflated before my very eyes. I wish I could go back in time and tell the younger, teenage me that her acne will eventually go away and her *ballooning* will calm itself down. Though it seems earth-shattering to not have perfect skin or the right curves, it truly isn't. I'd tell her that her focus isn't in the right place, and she needs to stop letting dissatisfaction with her appearance consume her. The frustration was mostly self-inflicted. I wish I could tell her that she needs to be more appreciative of her health and the strength of her body. She shouldn't dwell on the imperfections. And I wish she could listen—*truly listen*—to the friends who try to convince her the size of her clothing is just a number, and she doesn't need to torment herself by trying to squeeze into a size small. As long as it makes her look nice and feel comfortable, going up a size or two is perfectly fine.

Instead, I chose to sulk when I couldn't fit in the size I wanted and bought clothes that were too small, determined that one day I would fit in them. It was a ridiculous obsession. I hadn't realized no one really knew what size I wore, but they would *definitely* notice if something was too tight or didn't fit well. What was so attractive about fitting into a size zero, a size extra small, or a size small? (A friend jokingly pointed out it's a better deal to get larger-sized clothes because you pay the same price as a small!) Had I let the fashion industry brainwash me to allow such non-sense into my life? But somehow, I couldn't see past it. It was like I got sucked into this societal norm, ignored logic, and let it control my self-image. It made me waste so much of my time focusing on something so trivial.

I have heard many times it's what's inside that counts. But it didn't quite resonate with me until after I snapped out of that phase. While being bitter about my appearance, I couldn't appreciate the true meaning of *inner beauty*. I thought it was just fluff that tried to make unattractive people feel better about themselves.

Inner beauty doesn't suggest the person doesn't have outer beauty. It simply emphasizes there are so many ways a person can be beautiful. And beauty isn't only about being physically attractive. Have you met anyone who exudes love and acceptance to everyone alike? I know someone who greets everyone with genuine warmth. She makes you instantly feel better about yourself, feel wholeheartedly loved, and that you matter. When a homeless man walked into our church, she greeted him in the same manner. Most of us would likely turn away, wanting to distance ourselves from the preconceived filth and smell. But this friend of mine embraced this man fully in her usual loving way and gave him one of her beaming smiles.

"Welcome! It's so good to see you again!" she said as she looked him in the eye and addressed him by his first name.

I'll never forget that brief, monumental moment. It was clearly one of the highlights of his week. She saw him for who he was—a human being who was perhaps trying to find joy and a place in this world. And he was accepted just the way he was, despite being empty-handed and probably with not much to offer.

Thinking about my friend's behavior, I doubt she sulked endlessly about acne and not fitting in size zeros while growing up. Or perhaps she had her fair share of insecurities about her appearances but chose to focus her time and energy on doing good for others instead. She is so full of love and joy; they practically ooze out of her pores. And that is beauty beyond features and appearances. It's a kind of beauty that radiates and can change the world. It's beauty that matters.

My friend showed me that when we choose to saturate our lives with joy, we fixate less on what's wrong with our lives and instead focus more on how we can help spread this joy to others.

CHOOSING JOY
MY STORY

Life might throw curveballs at us sometimes, but if we learn to laugh along, it could make a world of difference.

My mom had cut my dad's hair for decades. And like most men, my dad needed a haircut every two or three weeks. So over time, my mom had given my dad many haircuts.

It was a sunny Saturday afternoon as they took the usual spot in the middle of their kitchen surrounded by tall windows. The sun beamed through as my mom lifted the hair clippers and started at the top of my dad's head. If you're familiar with the proper way to give a haircut, you'd normally start at the base of the head instead of at the top. But because my mom had become so familiar with my dad's hair, she had developed her own system that always delivered the style he liked.

What was different that day was my mom had accidentally forgotten to attach the trimming guard—the guard that keeps certain hair the same length. My mom pushed the clipper straight along the top of my dad's head and immediately let out a heart-stopping gasp. My dad's hair looked like someone just drove a lawnmower down the middle of his head, leaving a strip of barely-there, although quite neat, hair.

My mom stood there, jaw still wide open from realizing what she had just done.

And what did my dad do when he found out what had happened? *He laughed.*

Of all the reactions he could have chosen, he chose to laugh. He could have gotten angry, lost his temper, complained, laid blame, or badgered my mom on why this mistake shouldn't have happened because they'd done this *how many times?*

No. He chose to laugh. Dad chose joy over resentment.

By now, with that middle patch of hair so incredibly short, there were really no options left except to cut the rest of the hair to the same length.

And guess what? My dad *loved* it. He was proud to go out there in his new hairstyle, his new buzz cut. *The new buzz cut that his wife gave him.* He told people how they stumbled upon this hairstyle and how cool and light it felt to have shorter hair.

He did not dwell on the mistake or hang it over my mom's head. It became a funny memory in our family. For me, this was a very noble example of grace, of allowing people to make mistakes and going out of your way to help them not feel bad about it. And I saw the power of second chances. My dad happily continued to allow my mom to be his designated hairdresser.

It also showed me what a difference it can make to simply choose to laugh. When we learn to find humor in things, our lives can be so much brighter.

Being happy doesn't mean that everything is perfect. It means that you've decided to look beyond the imperfections.

—Gerard Way

TAKEAWAYS

- Count your blessings—there are indeed many!

- How you see yourself is important. Don't keep nit-picking on blemishes and imperfections. Focus on beauty that counts.

- Choose joy and choose to laugh. You are in control.

3

STAY TRUE TO YOURSELF

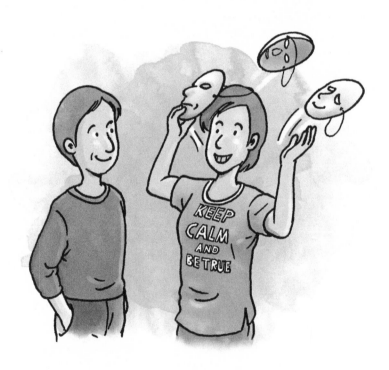

To be yourself in a world that is constantly trying to make you something else is the greatest accomplishment.

—Ralph Waldo Emerson

L et's face it, we all want to be liked. And why not? Being liked makes us feel good about ourselves. It makes us feel affirmed and worthy.

Our desire to be liked is evident in how much time and effort go into the selfies we take on our phones. It's as though, somehow, we *need* that approval on social media. We want others to take that extra pause to appreciate our *wowing* photo; we yearn for extra "likes."

Consider how much energy we invest into putting ourselves together to go out with our friends or on a date. We make sure our hair is perfect, our outfit is crisp, and our scent is appealing.

That need to be liked goes beyond our appearance. Sometimes, we change our personality traits or our behavior simply to fit in. When I asked people what life lessons they would share with their younger selves, a common theme was that they wished they had lived truer to themselves. There was typically a remorseful undertone as though they spent too much of their lives pretending to be someone else.

WHEN BEING COOL ISN'T ALL THAT COOL
ERNEST'S STORY

If I could go back in time, I would try harder to convince myself that being "cool" wasn't all that important. Everyone thought of me as the nice guy, the one they called on when they needed help. I should have realized that being the dependable one was a good thing. And I shouldn't have worked so hard to get rid of that label and create a "bad boy" image.

As I look back, it was so foolish of me to forcingly inject a slew of colorful swear words into my everyday language and to take up smoking because it seemed to attract the girls at the time. Why should I have been bothered to appeal to girls who were into bad boys anyway? And let's face it, it wasn't truly making me any more interesting of an individual.

I should have stayed true to myself and stood by the fact that my parents had raised me to be a decent person, help people without expecting anything in return, treat and speak to everyone with respect, and be kind. Why would I spend so much effort to go against that grain, especially when that grain pointed me in the right direction? My swearing initially sounded unnatural; it was obvious it was all an act. But that only motivated me to keep at it, to *practice* until it no longer sounded coerced, something so absolutely idiotic in hindsight. What did I gain in all this? I lost respect from those who mattered while fitting in with groups I really had no business being a part of in the first place.

THE PRICE TO FIT IN
JANE'S STORY

To say we weren't financially well-off is an understatement. My parents worked their fingers to the bone, trying to pay the mortgage and put food on the table. They sacrificed the little free time they had to work additional jobs to pay for our music lessons. We had no money left for unnecessary things like designer clothes. For years, I didn't know the difference. I had no concept of brands or fashion. Clothes were merely something you put on to go out, and it didn't matter what your outfit looked like or if your socks showed because your pants were too short. In the middle of high school, I learned there was a difference because my friends explicitly talked about it. They discussed designer jeans, designer backpacks, and designer shoes all the time. I learned of brands I had never known before. And while it didn't bother me that I didn't own any of these things, it soon made me feel inferior . . . deprived. I didn't blame my parents for not offering any of this expensive attire. They were trying their best. I am ashamed I guilted them into getting me designer jeans. I cannot recall how I had asked, but those jeans were a sacrifice my parents made even at discount store prices. They chose not to pay for *necessary* things to give me what I wanted.

As a proud owner of those designer jeans, I tried to stealthily show them off one Monday morning to two friends who had made such a big deal about them. Oh, and I thought I was so smart by standing at such an angle in front of them that they'd catch the logo. And I guess it worked because they did notice.

"Ooooh! You got new jeans! Where did you buy them from?"

Not expecting to be asked such a question, instead of honestly saying that they were from a discount store, I froze.

"Uh . . . I can't remember." That was my best answer in the moment.

I'm embarrassed to admit that even now. What kind of lame answer is "I can't remember?" when the purchase supposedly happened over the weekend?

I caught them smiling at each other before they went on to talk about something else.

The two seconds of attention were not worth the amount of thought I had put in to *finally* be able to own those jeans. They were certainly not worth adding more financial burden to my parents. These two girls were not even *friends* in the real sense. I allowed their materialism to impact my values. And in my attempt to try to be an equal, I was lying to myself, thinking one piece of clothing that remotely resembled what they wore would impress them. I wish I hadn't allowed their views to influence me so much. I wish I had been stronger.

TRUE FRIENDS SEE BEYOND THE SURFACE
AMY'S STORY

I had severe acne in my teens. Severe. They were painful to have and painful to see. I tried covering them up with makeup, but the foundation just looked caked on and almost called for more attention than if I had left them all red and full of puss. Every morning, I had to summon up

27

the courage to go to school and pretend no one could see my massive pimples. There were so many, and sometimes, it felt like they were starting to stack on top of each other from the diminishing vacant real estate on my face. My parents tried to persuade me this was just a phase, but I wasn't particularly keen on having my entire high school career with a dotted face. And who knew if it was even going to get better by the end of my teens? I had heard of adults having acne too.

Despite trying different remedies from topical creams to oral medications, nothing helped. "Perhaps it's all hormonal," one person suggested. But, so what if it was hormonal? Why did I have to be the one to live with it?

I wish I could give my younger self a great big hug and tell her she was beautiful. She wasn't beautiful *despite* the acne. She was, simply, beautiful. Period. The acne didn't take away her beauty; her concern with the acne made her fail to see her true beauty. Her friends didn't care that she didn't have a clear complexion. And had she been less obsessed with her skin, she would've noticed that a lot of other kids at her school battled the same problem. She was definitely not the only one with acne but thought she was and wallowed in it. I wish I could tell her she shouldn't have allowed herself to discount her worth due to what she considered a flaw in her appearance.

And yes, the acne did clear up.

THE COURAGE TO WALK
LESLIE'S STORY

My best friend was a bully. And somehow, I let her have this power over me that made me afraid of losing her friendship. So, I went along with her power trips, talked down to our peers, picked on them, and verbally abused them. Did I know it was wrong? Oh, you bet. But it wasn't enough to stop me from sticking around. Looking back, maybe I was afraid of becoming one of her victims. I had told myself that I wasn't truly involved as long as I stayed quiet while she picked on other people. I knew, in reality, I was still an accomplice.

Over time, as I saw the way her words tore people apart and broke down their confidence—which only made her feel better about herself—my conscience became increasingly troubled. So many times I challenged myself why I was allowing this to go on, knowing this *best* friend of mine wasn't really a friend. A good friend would help me to be a better person. She was far from that.

One day, I somehow found the courage to walk away. It might have been the realization that I did not want others to remember me this way, to let this define my school years. I told her the truth—how her bullying made me feel, how she had no right to talk down to anyone regardless of who they were, and how bad I felt for being a part of her actions. I risked being left with no friends. But I knew deep down that being a loner was better than being associated with someone so heartless and cruel.

29

I will never forget the way she looked at me as I said goodbye to our *friendship*. It was a mix of anger and disbelief. She tried to threaten me, but I stood my ground.

The days without friends were rough. It took a while to gain the trust of those my *friend* had bullied, but eventually, they let me in. There were weeks when I ate lunch alone, but I wasn't the only one—she ended up alone too. Without me by her side, she lost her power. Ultimately, I made new friends who were nice and caring; I looked up to them, and they made me want to be better. I never regretted breaking off a friendship that was dragging me down. So what would I tell my younger self? "I am so proud of your brave decision to walk away. It was not easy, but you knew it was the right thing to do. It's not easy to follow your heart sometimes, but you did it. I am proud of you."

Be what you are. This is the first step toward becoming better than you are.

—Julius Charles Hare

WEAR YOUR HEART ON YOUR SLEEVE
MARILYN'S STORY

I went in for my first job interview extremely nervous, unsure what to expect. People had advised that I study sample questions and answers, which I did, but at the same time, I was afraid that my answers would come out sounding overly rehearsed.

The interviewer greeted me with a warm smile and a firm handshake. My heart was pounding, and I tried to appear calm and collected. I really wanted this job.

Instead of going straight into my credentials, my interviewer simply asked me to tell him more about myself. I took the opportunity to highlight my academic qualifications and tried to pitch to him why I was the perfect candidate for the position. I consciously left out a big part of my life—my involvement at church, which in truth, taught me a lot of soft skills and a large part of how I define myself. I had wanted this job so much and didn't want to risk talking about faith and beliefs if it was too contentious of a topic.

My interviewer went on to tell me about himself. He began with his involvement at church. I smiled at the discovery that we shared the same faith, not because I thought it would help me get the job, but because I felt a more relatable connection with this potential employer. But my smile soon melted away as I realized how I had deliberately tried to hide something so important in my life. I had always considered my faith as being at the forefront of my identity. Why would it suddenly take a backseat at such an important milestone of my life?

31

This experience was a bit of a wake-up call in how I prioritized the various roles I have in my life. I am first and foremost a child of God, and everything else follows.

A MISTAKE CAN HURT MORE THAN YOURSELF
FRANCIS'S STORY

My parents had high hopes for me. I was the good boy in the family. My grandma called me her sweet boy, and we had a great relationship. She always made me feel special like I was somebody's favorite.

All that went out the window the day I mixed a little too much with the wrong crowd and started smoking. It wasn't so much the cigarettes themselves that were bad; it was the fact that this was the beginning of a downward spiral, a slow suicide. Smoking cigarettes turned to other substances, and soon after, I found myself doing drugs. It all happened so quickly. I don't remember actively deciding to try the different substances. It was more like a blur of events where one thing just led to another, and stopping was not an option.

And this all stemmed from an immense pressure to fit in, to have that sense of belonging. But I knew I shouldn't hang with these people. They didn't care for me but felt glorified in creating another addict.

Another addict. That's what I was. Another addict with a lifelong battle ahead, never quite sure when the urge would arise. Rehab took years. *Years.* These were years I wasn't ever going to get back. These *friends* certainly weren't going to give the years back to me. Were they around for support as I struggled every day to fight each temptation? No, all they offered was the easy way out, to turn back to drugs and feed the urge. Oh, and they weren't going to give it to me for free. I had to *pay* for them.

It ate me up that I was no longer my grandma's sweet boy. Though she never stopped calling me such, I'd like to think that it was because she was oblivious to all that went on in my secret life. But one time, I caught the way she looked at me, those tears in her eyes. Instantly, I knew. *She knew.* And yet she kept it that way, an unspoken understanding.

It pained me to know I disappointed her. But her tears told me her grief was in knowing the agony I was enduring, all that I had brought upon myself.

I believe she chose not to let it taint her love for me because she did not base her love upon how good or worthy I was of her love, but simply because I was her beloved grandson.

I wish I didn't let others have that much influence over my life choices. I wish I had understood that no one else would take responsibility for my actions and decisions. I wish I had known that, truly, the only person who had control over me was *me*.

TAKE CARE OF YOURSELF
PATTY'S STORY

I would have tried to understand myself more, to know what brought me joy instead of always trying to please people. When we are growing up and on the journey to find our identities, we often lose sight of what truly matters. I grew up in a family that was very much about obeying our parents. We had significant consequences if we did not follow orders. Soon, my siblings and I learned to manipulate the system and followed along for peacekeeping purposes only.

I married early to get away. My husband and I had children soon after, and I went from spending most of my time trying to please my parents to tending to my husband and our kids. The list of things to do for others was endless, and a lot of things went unnoticed. After a mental breakdown, I realized I never engaged in any self-care. I felt it was my job to be the perfect daughter, perfect wife, perfect mother, or at least bring myself to absolute exhaustion *trying* to be all of that. Unfortunately, I was under the delusion that women should be selfless beings, self-sacrificial, and always put others' needs before their own. I bought into the idea that focusing on my own happiness was selfish and inappropriate.

You cannot pour from an empty cup. It is so cliché to say but so true. If you are running on empty, there is only so much you can keep on giving to others. I wish I had learned earlier to seek what brought *me* real joy and find things that fed *me* happiness, which made *my* life worth living. Because when my heart is joyful, it will spread to how I serve others—in a manner full of joy instead of bitterness.

Let go of who you think you're supposed to be; embrace who you are.

—Brené Brown

34

TAKEAWAYS

- Peer pressure can be a powerful force that pushes us to be someone we are not. If this is hurting you and the people you care about, work hard to resist it if giving in to this pressure is turning you for the worse. Seek help; you don't need to fight it alone.

- Understand your values and how you identify yourself. Be bold about them; it's what makes you *you*.

- Being true to yourself also means taking care of yourself. Don't deny yourself love and care; they are imperative to your well-being.

4

MAKE TIME
FOR YOUR PASSION

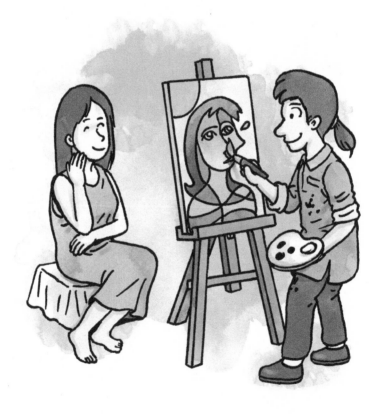

Twenty years from now you will be more disappointed by the things that you didn't do than by the ones you did do.

—Mark Twain

ake time for your passion. This might seem a little cliché, but given the premise of this book—life lessons from people on what they would tell their own younger selves—it's probably not surprising this is one of them. Many people look back and wish they had done something different in their lives—picked a different career, spent more time with family, learned a musical instrument, met more people, connected more with good friends, volunteered more, learned to draw, learned to dance, learned to sing, tried out different hobbies, and the list goes on. A lot of the time, they realized they wanted to explore an interest, but life got too busy, and they tucked it farther away until one day, it became the thing they never pursued.

Some people may not know their passion, have too many interests, are intimidated by the work, or feel afraid to start something new.

I believe that everyone has something they would *love* to do if they had all the time in the world. As life gets more hectic, it becomes more important to carve out the time, even if it's a mere ten minutes a day here and there. If you're not sure what your passion is or have a hard time choosing amongst a long list of things, the best first step may be to simply try. Pick something and invest a bit of time to see if it's what you want to pursue. It may resemble dating—you need to spend that time to know. If that particular interest doesn't appeal to you, try something else. Eventually, you'll figure it out.

If the work intimidates you, well, then that's a different story.

BE WILLING TO WORK HARD FOR IT

It may not always be easy to follow your passion. There could be a million reasons you give yourself why you shouldn't pursue it. If you have enough zeal about this passion of yours, if it makes you excited to get out of bed in the morning—assuming this passion does not cause anyone harm—then chase after it. Be ready for the journey, accept it will be easy on some days while other days leave you deflated, and fight that good fight. If you want something, you are going to have to work hard for it.

Some things have a more straightforward path than others. For example, if you want to learn a new skill—playing a musical instrument, knitting, baking, learning to play golf—there are classes you can take for those. And with the abundance of virtual classes, the options have become even more readily available. Just take the first step. Do some research and try it out. Then practice, practice, practice. You will only get better at it!

Effort pays off when it comes to your career. It also pays off to take the time to understand what you would consider a meaningful career. For some people, their life lesson was pursuing an appealing career catered to their passion and not what the mainstream told them they should do.

If you are exploring options for your career as a new graduate, it's not uncommon to not quite know what you want to do or how to figure out a path. Many people graduate from school without knowing exactly what to do. Internships are great as an exploratory tool. Competition for these opportunities can be fierce, so invest your time in identifying these opportunities (there are often more than we think) and then put your best foot forward. Employers are also trying to get something out of the internship, so show them what you have to offer that's different from everyone else. Don't underestimate the importance of showing up and being willing to deliver more than what's asked of you.

Some people argue it's best to let your good work speak for itself. Others say it's not enough to do good work; it's more important to promote your work so that it's prominent within the organization. However, I have seen the latter backfire more often than not. It's difficult to showcase your work humbly if you try to make sure people know about it. And humility is a virtue, not a weakness. Arrogance won't get you far; it could serve certain people for a while, but it could hurt you more than help you in the long run. If your work entails consistent quality, it will show for itself. People will recognize the person behind the work, the hardworking qualities, the talent. Find mentors and leaders who support you and have your back; let them be the ones who shine the spotlight on your work. And to do that, you do have to be prepared to work for it, so they know they can rely on you to deliver excellence.

Consider executive chefs. Think about the countless hours they work to improve their culinary techniques, perfecting dishes to ensure consistency, developing new recipes to continue introducing fresh signature dishes. Despite already being successful and owning popular restaurants, I believe these chefs don't stop sharpening their skills or innovating. Running a restaurant is very challenging; profits are thin, and the hours are long. Yet so many chefs push through to realize their dream to open a restaurant, and it's this perseverance—this grit—that gets them there. Even if they are anxious about the hard work, they find a way to overcome.

IT'S OKAY IF NO ONE ELSE HAS DONE THIS BEFORE

If uncharted territory holds you back from pursuing your passion and you haven't seen anyone else do it, then great! You could be a pioneer! Years ago, no one would have thought young kids could be making millions of dollars by having their own YouTube channel and creating content. Is there even an official occupation for this? These kids (and those who helped them along) probably didn't pause to wonder if there was a name for this job. It was something they enjoyed, so they tried it out. You may argue that these are kids—they don't have the pressure of making a living out of it—and that's true. If your passion isn't quite what you could see yourself turning into a full-time career, then try it out part-time first. Treat it as a serious hobby because a casual hobby is something we may continually put off when we are busy but really, when are we not busy? Dedicate time and energy consistently to this, foster it on the side, and perhaps one day it can replace your full-time job and salary.

DON'T WORK FOR MONEY; WORK TO BE BEST AT WHAT YOU DO

Money drives some people and lets that steer their career decisions. While it's important to choose an occupation that can support the lifestyle you and your family need or want, it's hard to work solely for money. Sooner or later, it loses meaning and purpose. If it's all about the money, it will become an endless chase, and you'd want more and more. There'd never be enough money for your job to give you a true sense of satisfaction. There has to be more than monetary gain to have true joy in what you do. You may know people who don't make a lot of money but are still content. It's usually because there are other aspects of their jobs that bring them true joy and meaning. It could be the ability to help others, to serve their community, or the opportunity to work with people with a similar mission.

Someone recently shared with me that it's not sustainable to work for money. If you strive to be the best at what you do, the results will follow. If you are a doctor and help people the best that you can, you could save many lives. Your delivery of quality care could also result in more prestigious pay. If you are a server at a restaurant and serve your customers the best that you know how, you may brighten someone's day. Great service tends to yield more generous tips and repeat business. If you are a teacher and teach to the best of your ability, your impact could very well ripple through generations to come.

DON'T FORGET TO HAVE FUN

If it stops being fun, it might be a sign for a change. Even within a company, there are many different positions you can test out to see if there is something else to find your passion. Life is too short to waste it. But life is certainly too long for us to be doing something we don't love. So, if what you do feels more like a drag and less that you're making an impact—in your life or someone else's—then be intentional in figuring out your possible next step.

I have heard of drastic career changes that helped people feel fulfilled once again.

David started with a political science undergraduate degree and worked several years in the field. It didn't bring him joy, and he felt the income wasn't worth the time he spent each day on something that left him increasingly dissatisfied. Deep down, he knew he was meant for more. From there, he went back to school to get a master's degree and found a new love in financial investments. He used that to launch into a career where he managed hundreds of millions of dollars for clients, thereby enabling a much better salary for himself. It took a lot of courage to pivot to a new career, but it made him so much more content that he knew it was well worth the risk and time to go back to school full-time.

Jared studied engineering in school more as a result of not knowing what else to choose. Engineering seemed promising of a safe, stable career path. However, he soon discovered a love for videography. As time went on, he realized he could capture moments in time that people wouldn't otherwise be able to capsulize. He learned there was so much he could be doing to serve others through his work. He went to school to get formally trained as a videographer and hasn't looked back. It wasn't easy switching careers; there was certainly doubt, especially in starting his own business. But the gratitude he received from his clients kept him encouraged to continue serving in a manner that aligned with his passion.

The most drastic career change I've heard of was a dentist who realized how much he hated working on people's teeth day in and day out and went on to become a farmer. How is that for following one's passion?

HIDDEN TALENT AND THE POWER
OF PERSEVERANCE
MY STORY

Many people claim they cannot draw, my mom and I included. About a year ago, my mom had the opportunity to participate in a virtual drawing class at her church. She signed up out of curiosity and joined a group of retirees on this weekly artistic journey, learning from scratch about various components and drawing techniques.

This was one of the first drawings my mom produced as a complete novice:

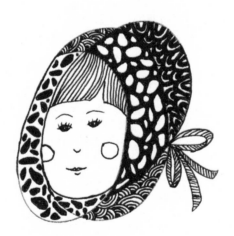

The concept was to make different free-hand patterns, then add in a doll face. She wasn't too pleased with how this turned out, but given she had just started learning to sketch a week or two prior, this was quite a job well done.

The teacher proceeded to assign pictures for the students to copy instead of doing things freehand.

By the fourth month, my mom was able to create this, simply by shading with a pencil on paper:

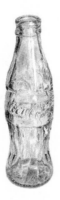

I was so impressed by the realism of this picture; I initially thought it was a photograph of a real glass bottle. The level of detail was nothing short of amazing.

It wasn't always smooth sailing. As much as my mom was encouraged by her progress and the compliments she received, there were times when she wanted to skip certain assignments because she believed she wasn't skilled enough to produce something of quality, especially since she hadn't been drawing for long.

There was one picture of an abandoned house that was especially challenging for her aging eyes. The details took her longer than usual to create the outlines. Her eraser became her new best friend. She set this aside time and again and contemplated giving up altogether. My mom eventually pushed herself to make progress, no matter how small. Though it took extra time, extra patience, and extra perseverance, she was ultimately able to complete this, six months after starting her art lessons:

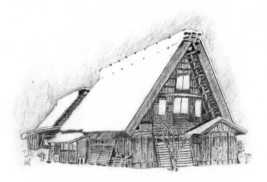

I believe this was a breakthrough for her. She proved to herself that there was really no limit to what she could draw, no matter how difficult it may look at first.

And a year after starting her journey as a budding artist, she was able to draw like this:

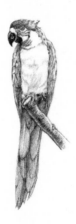

I am so proud to see the way my mom was able to develop her artistic abilities. She continues to pursue more and more challenging pieces; her determination is nothing short of inspiring.

LISTEN TO YOUR HEART
GRACE'S STORY

About five years after entering the workforce, I realized I had a knack for implementing project plans. When presented with a project end goal, it was natural for me to build out the plan and execute it well. With that, I was also mindful that I wasn't as much of a visionary. Strategizing at a high level wasn't my strong suit, but I was okay with that because of my enjoyment at execution. Plus, the more I worked at implementation, the better I got at it, and the better I got at it, the more I wanted to keep doing it.

Around that time, someone in the same company tried to recruit me to be on her team because she recognized my ability to execute. She was starting a new project and needed someone to fill that role. Ironically, around that same time, I had a conversation with an older friend who had significantly more work experience than I did. I had wondered out loud how to take my career to the next level. He advised mastering strategy development as a critical skill to get to the top. He said I needed to learn to be more of a thinker, to lead and provide direction, and that I had to start moving away from being a doer, an executor. He emphasized that the more others saw me as a doer, the harder it'd be to climb up the corporate ladder. I tried to explain my perspective, how much I truly enjoyed execution, bringing a project from concept to market. His final statement ultimately convinced me: "Remember that the C-Suite isn't just a bunch of doers. They strategize, they conceptualize, they create visions, and they lead. They do not focus on the day-to-day."

With that very fresh in my mind, I respectfully declined the job offer.

Years have gone by, and I wish I could have had a chance to tell my younger self it would have been quite all right to keep doing what she loved, what she was good at, where she continued to excel. I wish I could have told her that she'll have plenty of time to learn and practice creating strategies and leading a team. Her proven ability to get projects to launch with excellence paved her path to bigger things. The time she spent learning the building blocks will serve her and the people she works with in the future. It was time well-invested, not wasted. I would tell her that it was important she enjoyed what she was doing. She was making a difference, even though it may not have been apparent at the time. And she was fortunate to have found a passion that doubled up as a job and had an environment that fostered this passion and allowed her to blossom. Lastly, I would tell her not every career path needs to aim for the top. There are plenty of jobs that lead to meaningful careers without ever having a C title (not that there is anything wrong with C titles). It mattered more whether what she did was in tune with her heart.

A DANCER'S DREAM
KATIE'S STORY

It was my dream to become a dancer. I loved it so much and longed to dance professionally. My parents had a much more practical mindset about careers. They were quite sure artists typically starve. And dancers would have a similar outcome.

49

And so, they convinced me that instead of becoming a professional dancer, I should enjoy it on the side and pursue a different career, something that would put food on the table. They wanted the best for me, to ensure I had a bright future free of hardships, but their discouragement was crushing.

I couldn't figure out what else to study. It wouldn't have been wise to jump into something to pay bills but left me miserable for the rest of my life. So, I began to pick up small jobs to teach dancing. And that's what I ultimately ended up doing as a career. Because I was so busy trying to make ends meet while teaching, it consumed all my time and energy, and I eventually stopped pursuing dancing gigs that could have been stepping stones to something bigger.

If I could do it all over again, I would push my younger self to give it my all and follow my dream to become that professional dancer. Sure, my parents certainly disapproved, and they were not timid in sharing their minds. But this was my life. I owed it to myself to go after my dreams. Not everyone has a clear idea of what they want in life, so it deserves the pursuit when the vision is so vivid. Perhaps after giving it my absolute all, and if such a time came, I could have then resorted to becoming a dance teacher as the backup plan. I shouldn't have let myself lose sight of my passion for dancing professionally.

I would tell my younger self letting go of that dream so early on would leave her full of regrets and what-ifs. I'd tell her that she would end up instilling her dream in her students, but she should've been the one who went after it herself.

GOING AGAINST THE NORM
ANNIE'S STORY

I was career-oriented, very focused as I reached for the top. My path in the company was promising, and my contributions turned into one promotion after another.

Things felt different after I had my first child. I started feeling conflicted in how I split my time between work and family. Striking work-life balance was increasingly challenging. When my second child came along, the internal struggle only got worse. Every time my work bled into personal time, I felt this tremendous guilt, as though I was robbing from my family. And when I tried to draw a very firm boundary between work and family time, I felt I was no longer delivering my absolute best to my work, because there simply weren't enough hours in a day to do everything with excellence.

After discussions with my husband, we decided I'd take a break from work to focus on being a mother and a homemaker. It was far from what I had imagined for myself when I was young. I had never thought of myself as a stay-at-home mom, let alone voluntarily; it just didn't fit with the image I had of myself. We agreed if it didn't turn out to be what I wanted, I could go back to the workforce, and we'd figure out a way to get me out of the constant feelings of guilt.

Being a full-time stay-at-home mom took some adjustments at first. There were no work emails to tend to, no team meetings to lead, no executive presentations to prepare. Initially, it did make me feel unneeded. However, I was able to be present for my children, teaching them throughout the day. It was nice, and I learned to appreciate it more and more.

What I did not anticipate was somehow, as a homemaker, I felt less dignified. Somehow, it was as though I was *wasting* my talents. Although many of my friends had said they wished they could stop working so they could be home with their children, I felt judged when I turned it into my reality. It was as though not having to dash off to work and having only juvenile conversations throughout the day made me less relevant in society, less important.

It wasn't easy, but I eventually learned not to let others' opinions bother me. I was able to be there for my children physically, emotionally, and spiritually. I got to watch them grow up and not miss any more firsts. I could go back to be a working mother when the kids were more independent. It's a blessing for me to spend such dedicated time with my children. I knew my family was benefitting from my being a full-time mother, and it didn't matter what others thought.

Follow your passion. Nothing—not wealth, success, accolades, or fame—is worth spending a lifetime doing things you don't enjoy.

—Jonathan Sacks

TAKEAWAYS

- Life is short. Make time for your passion, time to do what brings you joy.

- Sometimes pursuing your passion can be challenging. Be willing to put in the effort, and you may be surprised by what you are able to accomplish.

- Don't forget to have fun!

5

YOUR WORDS ARE POWERFUL

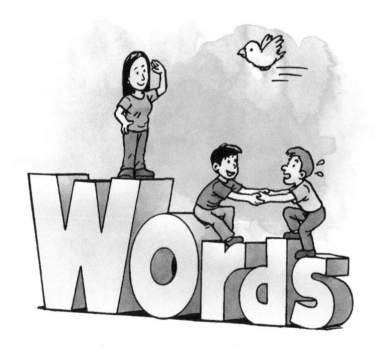

I've learned that people will forget what you said, people will forget what you did, but people will never forget how you made them feel.

—Maya Angelou

Words carry immeasurable power to lift someone up, to give them a boost of much-needed self-confidence. Or words can tear them down and instill self-doubt. It is an often-overlooked power because we use words every day at home, at school, at work, with our friends, strangers, and family. How often do we truly consider our words and evaluate the impact on the audience before we let them come tumbling out of our mouths?

We can probably think of multiple incidents in our lives where we have said something we wished we hadn't. And after we saw the hurt in the other person's eyes, we wished we could turn back time and take back those words.

BE RESPONSIBLE FOR YOUR WORDS

Consider how we treat our family. Often, we are more courteous with how we speak to our friends, even strangers, than with those at home—the ones who are closest to us. Perhaps there are more opportunities for conflict and friction at home, leading to more frustration and careless words. Or maybe we take our loved ones' forgiveness and understanding for granted. Either way, from my observation and perspective, this is common and happens frequently. I am just as guilty of this.

As much as we may try to justify talking back to our parents, insulting our siblings out of retaliation, or yelling at our kids as a form of discipline, there are better ways to respond. The key is to recognize when our anger is too escalated to suppress our cruel or unkind words—that is when we should simply step away. It's better than trying to take back hurtful words because as wonderful as it'd be, it's impossible to retract already spoken words. Like the analogy goes—you can hammer a bunch of nails into a piece of wood and take the nails back out, but the holes will always be there. There is no way for the piece of wood to revert to its original state. Likewise, our words leave lasting imprints on our loved ones' hearts, minds, and self-esteem. They may not remember the exact words and may forgive us before we even ask, but our actions likely caused avoidable pain and tears.

Why not save the best version of ourselves for those we love most?

A genuinely expressed "I am sorry" can do a lot of good. A heartfelt apology is powerful. We can't speak perfectly all the time. I certainly don't and continue to struggle to not let my moods take over my words. Emotions are real, but reconciliation is crucial. When you do or say something wrong, especially if it causes a lot of hurt, own up to it and apologize. An acknowledgment and apology have the power to renew hearts, including yours.

CHOOSE YOUR WORDS CAREFULLY
JACKIE'S STORY

Some time ago, I was asked to volunteer at a youth event. They needed a producer to help lead the event, and as I had experience in this area, they gave me the opportunity to help. A guest speaker, whom I shall call "Aaron," was invited to share a special message with the students.

I held a meeting with the key players, including Aaron, about an hour before the event to go over all the details and ensure everyone understood the flow of the night. I tried to lead the meeting efficiently since there wasn't a lot of time to make changes or rehash things. We had to get it right the first time around.

Everyone had a copy of the agenda in their hands. As I walked through the rundown with the team, I made sure to call out, in great detail, what each person needed to remember, their specific cues, and so forth. Everything was carefully written out on physical paper in the attempt to make the event truly failproof. Given this was my only chance to prepare everyone simultaneously, it was critical they remembered their cues, what they had to cover, and their transitions to the next segment.

Glancing at my watch again and again, I talked through each section. Time was ticking away, and the pressure of wrapping up my meeting in time intensified by the second.

"And where do I come in?" Aaron suddenly piped up.

Instantly, I felt irritation bubble up inside of me. His name was in the next section, clearly written in bolded letters, and it was *less than two inches below* the part we were talking through at that moment.

"It's where it says 'Guest Speaker (Aaron) enter with mic from stage left. Start speech.' Right here." I held up my paper, and with a slight tap of my finger, pointed to the exact location on my paper. Despite my ability to keep a smile on my face, I heard an edge in my voice, and it was obvious my response was condescending and signaled impatience.

"Oh, I see," Aaron said quietly with a genuine smile. "Thank you."

I continued talking through the rest of the agenda, dismissed the team, and moved on to the rest of my preparation work.

The event soon started. Everything went smoothly according to the agenda. Then, it was Aaron's turn to take the stage. He introduced himself and explained why he was there that night. "It's possible to overcome life's obstacles. I know because I had to overcome my biggest challenge—dyslexia."

Aaron had dyslexia.

I froze. It felt like someone had punched me in the stomach. However, it was probably nothing compared to the sting—the invisible slap—my words had inflicted earlier. My brusque words and unnecessary gesture of holding up the agenda, pointing to his *clearly written* name—for those of us who could read—but not clearly legible for those with dyslexia.

It wasn't a lack of attention or an attempt to deliberately cause trouble, and it wasn't him being *too lazy* to scan the rest of the agenda. He simply couldn't read words like the rest of us could.

I never had a chance to apologize to Aaron because he left immediately after his speech that night.

This incident happened about ten years ago. Although it has been *almost a decade* since, I still recall it like it was yesterday. No doubt Aaron had probably encountered similar treatment from others as a result of his disability. Perhaps he was accustomed to insensitive remarks, making it pointless for him to explain himself that night. What mattered to me, however, was how poorly I had treated him, and I was not proud of my actions.

I hope Aaron has already long forgotten about this and that my actions didn't leave a scar. More importantly, I hope he has already long forgiven me for it. But I guess I'll never know.

And unfortunately, such is life. Sometimes, we take opportunities for granted and somehow assume we will have the chance to undo, redo, apologize, or seek forgiveness, but that isn't always the case. The truth is, sometimes we only get one shot.

Would we choose our words more carefully if it's the *absolute* last time we get to speak to that person?

Imagine all the other reactions I could have had. What if I had kindly asked him to hold his question for another thirty seconds because his section was next. I could have simply answered his question without being a smart mouth. Better yet, I could have treated him respectfully like a guest, which he was. And what if I had genuinely thanked him for trying to thoroughly understand his part? At the end of the day, that was why he had asked, right? He was trying to make sure he did what he could to help us execute the event flawlessly.

SOME WORDS ARE BETTER LEFT UNSPOKEN
ANNABELLE'S STORY

During a subway ride from work one day, I observed two friends, likely in their twenties, who had bumped into each other and were overjoyed by the opportunity to chat during the long commute. They appeared to be more than acquaintances but perhaps hadn't seen each other in months. They quickly launched into catch-up mode, going from topic to topic, talking fast and laughing a lot, as though fearing they would run out of time.

I went back to reading my book until I suddenly heard one of them say, "Oh, but you know, that's such a controversial subject."

"What does *controversial* mean?" she asked matter-of-factly.

"You don't know what controversial means?" he responded, raising an eyebrow.

She paused slightly and shifted her body uncomfortably. "No."

"Uh . . . it's like something that a lot of people may not agree with."

As an outsider, their sudden lack of enthusiasm, frowns, and serious eyes all showed that the rest of their conversation was not the same. Somehow, the way he threw in that question, almost doubting her intelligence, changed things. Her guard went up as though protecting herself from further judgment, to prevent any more opportunities to feel inferior, to feel *dumb*. That one *simple* question likely did some damage that day for both her self-esteem and their friendship. Sure, "controversial" might not be a word most people would consider difficult, but she didn't know the

61

meaning, plain and simple. He didn't need to make it sound so out-of-the-ordinary, so shocking. True friends help each other grow, even with vocabulary. And they should do it without making the other person feel incapable or weak.

Be mindful when it comes to your words. A string of some that don't mean much to you, may stick with someone else for a lifetime.

—Rachel Wolchin

TAKEAWAYS

- Your words matter; use them carefully.

- Let the words you speak build people up and not tear them down.

- Apologies are necessary for healthy relationships. Genuinely say you're sorry when you have done something wrong.

6

RESTRAIN YOUR PRIDE

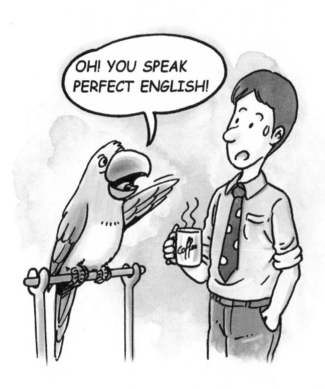

You learn nothing from your life if you think you are right all the time.

—Toby McKeehan (a.k.a. TobyMac)

When things are going well, it's easy to fall into the trap of thinking we deserve that when, in fact, it may not have been us who created the favorable circumstances. It's also easy to blame other factors when things are not going well for us instead of assuming responsibility.

I worked with someone who used to mock other employees who were immigrants and couldn't speak perfect English. Gary would imitate their accents to get a good laugh. Until one day, one of his friends finally spoke up about it. He reminded Gary the only reason these people couldn't speak English well was that it wasn't their first language, and Gary's parents were immigrants and also couldn't speak perfect English. Gary *could* speak fluent English because his parents took the brunt of the immigration hardship, moved to another country, and learned a different language mid-life. Gary had an easy life, reaping the benefits of his parents' hard, tireless work. This friend also reminded Gary that these immigrants were trying to speak English to carry out their job and respect their colleagues. After that, Gary no longer poked fun about this language difference.

Don't be prideful about things you did nothing to earn just because you were born into a better situation than others. Don't be boastful of the things your parents, grandparents, or ancestors earned through hard work and sacrifices. You're a beneficiary. That doesn't come with a right to flaunt or brag.

Learn to be comfortable that you may not have all the answers and may not be the smartest person in the room. You do not need to strive to be the smartest. Use that as motivation to push yourself to grow.

Don't be arrogant about status.

AN ENLIGHTENING REALIZATION
JACOB'S STORY

I had some lucky breaks early in my career. Soon, I found myself as the youngest person with my work title and scope of responsibilities in a large company, a reserved parking spot and luxury car to park in it, and weekly meetings with the C-Suite. At first, I took pride in all these things. They symbolized a significant accomplishment to me. I felt important. I'm glad I never verbalized how proud I was about all that because as I got older, my perspective changed. My achievement was less an indication of my talents and more how much faith the company had in me. They were willing to take a chance with my lack of experience. As the youngest in the board room, it may have been something to be proud of, but my more mature side recognized that it also meant I was the least seasoned person in the room. Once I could discern that difference, I focused less on how much I had come along and more on how much farther I had to go. It wasn't that I diminished what I had accomplished to date. I continued to be grateful for the recognition my company gave me. What changed was that I no longer viewed myself as that big of a deal. Being a young executive meant the company had entrusted me with more responsibilities than others my age, but I still had much to learn.

TRANSFORMED LEADERSHIP
ANDREW'S STORY

A failing department hired me to help transform and save an imploding company. With that responsibility and recognition for my abilities, I walked into the job full of confidence, and my nose was a little too high in the air. I wish I could go back in time and smack my younger self a few times so he could see that displaying such arrogance wasn't going to get him anywhere. You cannot walk into a new company and try to get people's buy-in by convincing them you have all the answers. Effective leadership and cockiness don't mix well. It is impossible to gain support by making people feel stupid or by talking to them like they can't keep up with you. My initial approach damaged a lot of relationships. Some people outright said they could never be paid enough money to work for me again.

It took me years to learn and evolve to true servant leadership. I figured out I had to cater to others' learning and working styles and not for them to conform to mine. I realized my role as a leader was to serve and help remove obstacles for my team to perform at their best. I finally understood that a lot of times all my team needed was my support, encouragement, and belief in them. And it all starts with genuine humility. Jokingly, I told people I worked *for* *them*, not the reverse. As much of a joke as it was, that was my real approach to leading a team. I was there to serve them. Their needs and best interests were above my own.

Fortunate for me, the people I offended were gracious. They gave me a second chance to repair our relationships and to show them I was capable of change. They gave me another shot at doing what they hired me to do—to transform a broken company. I just hadn't realized that part of what needed significant transformation was me.

DON'T FORGET WHERE YOU CAME FROM
BRITTANY'S STORY

I had the privilege of working with an intern whose ethnicity and culture were different from mine. There was a bit of a language barrier, more because of contextual difference rather than fluency. I hired him because he came across as knowledgeable, hardworking, and dedicated. He was over-qualified to be an intern, but he needed a foot in the door.

On a particular day as he returned from break, I asked whether he had a good lunch. Honestly, I asked the question more out of habit as a way to exchange pleasantries like, "How are you?" and "I am fine." Perhaps it was due to the cultural difference, but his honest answer caught me by surprise.

"I didn't eat lunch."

Not quite knowing what to say after that, I blurted out, "Oh? How come?" I silently scolded myself for belaboring the conversation.

I was glad I asked.

"I only have one meal a day," he explained. "I'll eat when I get home."

At that time, I hadn't met anyone who only ate once a day. He might have picked up the cue of my raised eyebrows, for he automatically continued.

"I am used to not eating all the time. Back home, my brothers and I took turns eating on alternate days."

I am pretty sure my jaw dropped all the way open.

Took turns eating on alternate days?!

And that was this gentleman's reality—growing up eating on select days throughout the week. His parents did not have enough food to feed all their children at every meal and had to ration it among their kids.

It was extremely humbling. I could not fathom not having a full belly regularly.

This gentleman found a full-time job at another company after his internship ended. I didn't hear from him until a few years later, when a headhunter reached out to me for a reference. It was for a high-ranked position within a high-profile organization. I was proud to see the progress he had made in such a short time, leaning on his effort and determination. His subsequent call told me that he got the job. He thanked me wholeheartedly, not only for my advocacy that facilitated his hiring but for giving the internship to start him on a good path—the internship he was overqualified for. A few years later, he continued to move on up and is doing very well professionally. He once again thanked me for helping him advance through his career, giving me more credit than I deserved. Despite his success, he remained humble and grateful.

Humility is not thinking less of yourself, but thinking of yourself less.

—C.W. Lewis

TAKEAWAYS

- If those who came before you paved the way for your success, be grateful. Alternatively, if you started with nothing and found success through hard work, never forget where you came from.

- Don't strive to be the smartest person in the room nor to have all the answers. Leave space for yourself to learn and grow.

- Leading with humility can make a world of difference.

7

SET GOALS

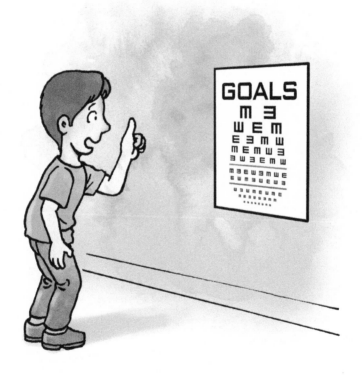

Setting goals is the first step in turning the invisible into the visible.

—Tony Robbins

No matter how big or small, goals matter. They keep us from simply drifting along, letting life steer us wherever, whenever, however. Goals act as a compass to guide us on our journey.

Without goals, life would lack purpose. We need a clear definition and plan to pinpoint our destination.

How would we know how to best spend our time without goals? How would we know when to say yes and when to say no? Without goals, we'd operate in a passive mode; we'd fall into a meaningless type of busyness. If we have a clear idea of what we want to accomplish, we can more easily determine what is worth our time and what is not.

Some people are more natural at goal setting than others. I have observed people who don't explicitly set goals, but somehow, their actions make the journey toward their goal obvious; there is a clear blueprint in their mind on how to get there.

Others may not have the knack for creating goals, but because they recognize the importance of goal-setting, they consciously develop habits centered around their dreams and aspirations.

And some people take things one day at a time, with no vision of where they are going.

Don't just *wing it* in life; that's hardly ever a good strategy to approach any task or important component of life. Don't let yourself get to the end of your life only to realize that *winging it* didn't pan out well.

Define what success looks like to you. And success doesn't have to be defined by wealth or fame. Success can be building meaningful, lasting relationships, maintaining good health, raising independent children who are a positive contribution to their community, being able to take care of your aging parents, and the list goes on. Success depends on what matters to you, but it needs to be clearly defined.

Even if you haven't been setting goals for yourself, it's better now than never. Understanding that goals are important is a good first step. Next, start taking action and start thinking! If you don't know how to get started, here is some guidance:

FOLLOW THE S.M.A.R.T. RULES

S.M.A.R.T. is a simple tool to facilitate your goal setting. Since so many New Year's resolutions are about physical fitness, let's use that as an example. Let's say my overall desire is to be in better health.

S – Specific. Pick something that isn't ambiguous or vague. For example, it'd be better not to say, "I want to be healthier" or "I want to be skinnier." Instead, find something more specific. How about: "I will cut down my intake of processed sugars to no more than twice a week" or "I will lose two inches off my waist" or "I will train to run a marathon in twelve months."

M – Measurable. When something isn't measurable, it's hard to say whether you succeeded or not. "I want to be more physically active" isn't helpful because *more* isn't measurable. Rather, opt for something black and white. If you opt for "I will exercise more" as a goal, would doing ten push-ups count? By defining what you will be able to do, such as reducing the waistline by two inches or being able to run a certain distance by a specific date, you can easily identify whether you have accomplished the goal.

A – Attainable. Goals should challenge you but not discourage you before you even start. Setting realistic goals helps. However, don't make it so easy that it requires little effort. Give yourself a stretch so you can feel proud for having put in the hard work. If you are only starting to work out, it may not be realistic to run a marathon in a month or two. Perhaps start with a 5K or 10K in that same time frame. Once you accomplish that, it'd be easier—and more attainable—to add more distance from there.

R – Relevant. Your goals should align with your values and overarching direction to carry meaning, and they should keep you motivated. Essentially, the goal should be important to help you clearly understand whether it's time well-invested. In our example, if physical health is important to you and your loved ones, then the goal for better fitness is relevant. Your goal should align with your *why*.

T – Time-bound. This is critical. Establishing a timeline as to when to achieve this goal gives you set boundaries. Boundaries are important because they motivate us to perform at our best. It would be pointless to strive for better health but not define a deadline. It would be futile to say, "I want to be able to run a marathon"—there would be little drive to get started. If you are twenty-five now and still haven't run that marathon by age fifty, does that mean you haven't met the goal, or are you simply still working toward the goal? Conversely, if you tell yourself, "I want to be able to run a marathon in twelve months," then you know you need to start training. There is now a fire within you to move and take action.

Having defined time frames work hand-in-hand with the measurable aspect of goal setting. Because your goals are specific, there is really no gray area to allow for negotiations on whether you finished. If you want to be crushing your goals, it's important to be honest with yourself and don't leave room for excuses or sliding targets.

If you aim for nothing, you'll hit it every time.

—Unknown

START BIG AND WORK YOUR WAY DOWN

Identify a major goal you would like to achieve. Is there a particular skill set you would like to master, an industry you'd like to pursue, or a specific occupation you would like for your career? Would you like to save for a down payment for a house or have enough money for your dream vacation?

Once you have identified your big goal, break it down into smaller segments. The milestones will seem less overwhelming, will allow you to celebrate the small wins, and will keep you motivated to continue pushing forward. Small steps accumulate to achieving great things.

Let's use the example of saving for a dream vacation since vacations are fun. First, let's identify where we want to go. I would love to go back to the African safari, so let's use that for our illustration.

1. Research the total cost of the trip—flights, accommodations, tours, and excursions. Add those up. Let's say it's $5,000. (Don't freak out. I'm using fake numbers, but vacations *can* get expensive!)

2. Estimate daily expenses such as meals (if not covered by the tours), shopping, tips, etc. For simplicity, let's use $100 per day for a nice, round number. For a ten-day trip, that's another $1,000.

3. So, now you know you need $6,000 for your trip. That's your *big* goal.

4. Next, estimate when you may want to go on this trip. How about in two years? This tells you that in twenty-four months, you need to have saved $6,000. That works out to saving $250 each month.

(Note: I used twenty-four months for illustrative purposes only to simplify the calculations. If your trip is truly in twenty-four months, you may need to spend the money earlier than that (for example, booking the flights), so your timeline should be according to when you need to spend the savings versus when you will be making the trip.)

Breaking your goal down into smaller, digestible chunks can effectively help you toward success. It can keep you from feeling so overwhelmed you may not even want to attempt the first step.

DEVISE A PLAN TO ACHIEVE YOUR GOAL

Similar to determining the route to get to your destination, you'll need a good plan to help you achieve your goals. Not all plans are equal; some get you faster to your goals, and some involve detours. However, it's impossible without a plan. When in a foreign country, you may agree that to visit attractions, you wouldn't wander aimlessly, hoping to stumble upon those places *eventually*. No, a better approach would be to plot out your routes so you can see those places before it's time to hop on your flight home.

> *People with goals succeed because they know where they're going.*
>
> —Earl Nightingale

Let's go back to our example above on saving money for your trip to Africa. Once you know you need to save $250 *every month*, you'll need to figure out how to get there.

1. Take a good look at your monthly cash inflow and out-flow and determine where you can make adjustments. You may find that you'll need to spend less somewhere or make sacrifices. Perhaps it's streamlining in multiple areas. Try not to shave it from your long-term savings. Start by making near-term adjustments first.

2. It might help to create a visual aid to track your prog-ress. Find an app that enables you to keep track, or, for a more encouraging, in-your-face visual, create a chart on a poster board (like a thermometer image), so you can see how your savings are accumulating. I

have seen people track this on their bathroom mirror, so it's front and center. You see it when you wake up in the morning and before you go to bed at night. If tempted to spend that money, create a bank account and transfer the money out of your regular account, so the money is out of reach and protected.

3. If you cannot set aside $250 per month no matter how hard you try, then evaluate your options. Perhaps there is a way for you to increase your income. Pick up a side job or find a project to earn some extra cash. That might help you get to your goal even faster. If your circumstances make it unfeasible to squeeze out that spare time to generate a separate income, another option would be adjusting your timeline accordingly. Perhaps this is a trip further down the road instead of two years. And that's okay! It would still be worth saving. Or select a different destination so you can still have a trip to look forward to in two years.

ACCOUNTABILITY PARTNERS

We need to hold ourselves accountable to our goals. When factors are within our control, this is very important because it's easy to let things slide—push out the timeline and reduce the scope—when no one is checking on you. You may even scrap the whole goal and try to start fresh! So, find ways to hold yourself accountable. Write it down. Display it where it is visible every day. Post it on social media so it's public. Break the plan down to actions you need to take to keep you on track. Look at your progress regularly to understand whether your pace gets you to your goal in the time frame you have set for yourself.

Having an accountability partner can help tremendously. Find someone to report your progress to regularly that can help you move toward your goal. You need someone you would be honest with and not hide the truth of your development and struggles. This is someone who can collaborate with you to break down these obstacles to keep you going forward. They will encourage you but not let you off easily. They will be your cheerleader.

Only postpone your deadline as a last resort; even if you encounter hurdles that push you back, find ways to compensate for the time loss; otherwise, you might go too easy on yourself. Challenge and stretch yourself and thrive.

WHEN EVERY SMALL STEP COUNTS
MY STORY

I have friends who are avid readers, and I was one, too, when I was single and childless. Once parenthood started, it became a struggle to find time to read. Yet I had observed people with similar busy lifestyles (or perhaps even more) manage to read a lot. I also noticed they typically had concrete goals in the number of books they planned to read each year. Not *hope* to read but *plan* to read. Twenty-four books in a year seems like a common objective. At first, that felt like a very intimidating task when there is so much happening with work, family, and life in general. After all, it's not like I am on summer vacation where I can lounge on a beach and read for leisure.

I let this seemingly impossible undertaking remain on my wish list, brushing it off as something my busy schedule couldn't possibly afford at this stage of my life. It was easy to devise convincing excuses to justify why I shouldn't even try to achieve this. I mean, come on, twenty-four books meant two books every month. That's one whole book every two weeks. And with the number so out of reach, I let myself be comfortable with a laughably small goal instead. If twenty-four is so hard, let's start with at least one book a year.

As a new year's resolution that year, I picked up a business book on leadership. I subconsciously noticed I was reading at a pace of ten pages in fifteen minutes, which equated to forty pages every hour. For whatever reason, I started to do some quick calculations. The book had 275 pages. That meant I could read the entire book in less than seven hours. Guess what that looks like when spread over two weeks? A half-hour each day. I could finish one book in two weeks by reading merely thirty minutes a day.

Instantly, a lightbulb went on in my head. Reading twenty-four books in a year no longer seemed so unattainable after all. Sure, some books are longer, and some may be heavier in substance and require a slower pace, but some books are also shorter and easier to read. In essence, reading twenty-four books in twelve months—even for a busy working mother with two young children, a full-time job, and a manuscript to complete—is totally doable!

From there, I set out to read at least a little every day. Some days I merely read ten pages; other days, I managed to squeeze in a little more. By the end of the first month of my revelation, I was already halfway through my third book.

If not for breaking things down into bite-sized chunks (or daily objectives), I may still have aimed for one book a year.

Likewise, in our vacation budget example, coming up with $6,000 can feel so daunting, and you may tell yourself not to bother trying. *Guess I'll only go to Africa if one day I win the lottery.* However, once you break it down to $250 per month (or less, if you spread it out over a longer time frame), it becomes much more realistic.

WORK HARD FOR SOMETHING TO BE PROUD OF
MANDY'S STORY

The annual marathon was coming up in several months. I usually register early to take advantage of the early bird rates. Each year, my goal is to simply complete the race because that is already a major accomplishment. And every year, I'd consistently finish it in roughly the same time.

One particular year, I wanted to do more than merely finish. I decided to push myself to complete the marathon at a much quicker time. This would be an attainable goal, but it would make me work harder. *Much harder.*

The thought of crossing that finish line with my new goal time on the big clock made me smile. It also made me nervous—how was I going to make it happen?

With the goal in mind, I set out to do some serious planning. First, the work-back schedule. What speed did I need to achieve by what time to have a chance at achieving my goal on the day of the marathon?

I had my training days with my running group penciled into my calendar. This was a major part of enabling success because it's tough to run for hours alone on a regular basis.

If I wanted to hit my goal, I had to stick with a strict regimen for at least the three months prior to the main event. I focused extra hard at work to ensure I could leave on time each day to head straight to running.

After a few weeks, I realized I wasn't training frequently enough with my running group and risked not hitting my goal time. I didn't want to choose to give up, though that could have been an option. So, I chose to train harder for that goal by evaluating my options.

A friend referred me to a coach who helped to guide me in all aspects, from improving my running technique to giving me tips on what to wear. There was a secret to every second I wanted to gain.

I also started running independently and with my group to condition my body more, building it up for longer and longer distances.

Later, my coach did another assessment and revealed my goal was still too much of a stretch. I needed more speed. Marathons are a tricky thing. Most people think it's all about endurance, and stamina is a large part of it, but you also need to strategically sustain a certain speed for each mile if you want to complete the 26.2 miles within a specific time. And 26.2 miles is a long way to travel on foot, even for walking, let alone running.

One more option to consider was to shed some weight so I could increase my speed. There truly is a science behind it. For each fewer pound you carry on you while you run, you should be able to gain so many seconds in speed.

Losing weight is not easy when you need to feed your body at the same time to give it the energy, strength, and endurance to do the miles on a daily basis. I also had to be stricter about eliminating junk food. Junk food slows the body down and contributes to fat-building, so including it to my diet would counter what I was trying to accomplish. During this phase, I leaned on my coach even more. It's hard to stay on track by yourself. My coach was not only my teacher but also my cheerleader.

The day of the marathon arrived quickly. I'm happy to share I finished slightly *under* my goal time. The sense of pride and accomplishment as I crossed that line, seeing my time on the clock, left me speechless. It was like a dream becoming a reality. I'd bet I was beaming toward the sea of strange faces surrounding the finish line.

The hard work was well worth it. What made me the proudest was I allowed myself to dream big, and I did not give up. It was hard to push my feet to keep pounding the pavement, to ignore the burn, to overcome the pain. Having people to lean on throughout the process made it less daunting, less like the unattainable dream. I may have been able to do it on my own, but having people rally around my goal, to help me stay focused, talk me out of quitting, and encourage me along the way made a world of difference. It helped me to cross the finish line in less time than I'd thought possible.

The greater danger for most of us is not that our aim is too high and we miss it, but that it is too low and we reach it.

—Michelangelo

TAKEAWAYS

- It's important to set goals in life so you know where you are going. Use the S.M.A.R.T. framework to help you define your goals.

- Break big goals down into smaller goals to help you stay encouraged and on track.

- Be accountable. If it's challenging to hold yourself accountable, seek a supportive accountability partner to assist you on your journey.

8

PAUSE TO REFLECT

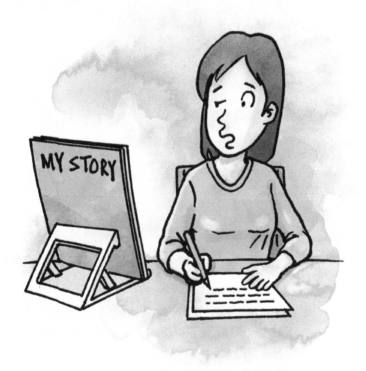

Without reflection, we go blindly on our way, creating more unintended consequences, and failing to achieve anything useful.

—Margaret J. Wheatley

Many of us may not be completely content with life, and others may be outright dissatisfied, but we choose to accept and tolerate that reality.

If you don't like your current path, then try to change it. It's almost silly to not try to do *something* to change course. Don't stay on the path merely because it's the easiest. You'll likely come to a point where you regret sticking with the easy.

Reflection forces us to take a good look at where we came from, how far we have come, and how much we have grown. At the same time, it could give us a realistic view of how much we have come short of our goals or steered off path. It could also make us realize the path we are on will not land us where we ultimately want to be and that we need to do something about it—*right now*. A lot of people fail to make this realization because they don't take the time to reflect. Or they may not be doing it often enough.

Imagine you are writing your autobiography—would you be pleased with your story?

Imagine you have passed away. Would your eulogy make you proud as the legacy you're leaving behind? What are others going to remember about you? How did others view you, and what did you mean to them? Who would be at your funeral? These are people whose lives you will have touched in some ways throughout your life. Are there many, or would the room be empty? Once in a while, take the time to give this some thought. No one knows exactly how long they will live. Almost everyone would expect to live a relatively long life. To die young is a tragedy. I know three young men who died from motorcycle crashes in their early twenties. They all went out one particular day, expecting to come home. Their family said bye to them, not knowing it would be the last goodbye. It's cliché to say *live each day as though it's your last*. For many of us, that could mean we'd quit our jobs and live however we choose until our very last day. But without truly *knowing* what day is our last, it would be irresponsible to quit our jobs and live carelessly. That expression is more to encourage us to live each day to its fullest so that even on our last day, we would not have regrets.

REFLECTION ISN'T ALL ABOUT REGRETS

Reflection isn't simply looking back, thinking: *What if* and *if only* and *I wish I had* and *I wish I hadn't*.

Reflection is a great tool for mentally and physically mapping out our current course and seeing where we'd land if we were to stay on the same path, doing the same thing day in, day out. Without external factors to cause a change in direction, you can easily imagine where you'd end up. And whether that picture makes you happy or afraid is a good indication of whether you should be doing something differently.

If you are already years into your career, unless you purposefully make a change, you will likely do the same thing until the day you retire. Usually, you do not stumble into a new career, especially if what you do today is very specialized. You may experience career development, for example, growing into a leadership role, but if you don't make at least some effort to change, it isn't going to happen.

Job changes take work. A recruiter may knock on your door based on your credentials, but unless you go through the interviewing and evaluation process, which takes work on your end, you won't automatically be handed the job. So, if you are resistant to change and choose to shut the door on the opportunity before putting in the effort to learn about the new employer, the industry, their challenges, and where you can help them grow, you will likely stay put exactly where you are. And if you're okay with that, then it's great you're doing something you find fulfilling and rewarding. If you're not okay staying where you are, you need to put in the effort to contribute to the change, whatever the cost.

So, while reflection isn't only about looking back and being bogged down with regrets, it can facilitate in identifying potential regrets in the future. It helps you look back *and forward* so you can chart out a life that's worth living for you and your loved ones.

REFLECT TO GET BACK ON TRACK

Some key reflections can lead us to make drastic decisions and have a major impact on our future. For example, when we recognize our draining, dead-end job will no longer serve us well, we find a new job or a new career. That is bigger than things like recognizing declining dietary habits and physical activity, and emerging body aches and pains. When you chart out your course and realize the endpoint of where you're heading isn't where you want to be, you'd want to make the proper corrections. Even a one-degree shift in your trajectory can land you somewhere entirely different by the end of your journey.

And there are annual changes. A lot of people gravitate toward new year's resolutions. It seems to be the perfect time to commit to change—a new year signals a new beginning, a fresh start. So, what better time to impose changes?

Yet many people only manage to stick with their new year's resolutions for the first month or two before they fall off the wagon. Then, they try again the following year. You can argue that it's the lack of commitment, but it's likely more than that. Building a new habit takes time, effort, and energy. The earlier you create good habits, the easier it'll be as you progress through life. But developing new habits during mid-life can be challenging.

The New Year's Eve countdown and fireworks can be exciting and celebratory in nature, but once they fizzle out (no pun intended), you need those fireworks to keep momentum with your new year's resolutions. So, when you suddenly find yourself no longer going to the gym, what would you do? First, don't sweep it under the rug and tell yourself, *I'll try again next year.* No, you can do better than that! Reflect on what held you back from going to the gym. Was it a particularly busy week? Was it due to poor planning? If yes, then plan and get back on track. Schedule the gym time into your calendar and protect it. Perhaps you need to reduce the duration of your workouts temporarily, say, changing it from an hour to a half-hour session. That might be easier to stick with, and you can build from there.

Perhaps you were getting bored with your exercise. If you're not sure, then try to change that and see if you find your motivation. Sometimes, simply changing the scenery can make a big difference.

Or perhaps you need a workout buddy to be a source of encouragement and accountability.

Taking this pause to assess your past week or month can do wonders. It allows you to correct veering off-path sooner and requires less work to get back on track. Someone who has stopped working out for three years would have a much harder time restarting *and sustaining* a regular workout schedule than someone who lacks motivation for a week but proactively corrects that. The latter can jump right back, practically without missing a beat. The former would need much more effort to establish a new routine then work even harder to keep it.

So, push back from the urge to let yourself fall off the wagon completely. If you need a break, then schedule time for that, but have a fixed date to get back.

REFLECT TO IMPROVE

Reflection can also help us maintain relationships. After an argument with a loved one, while still at the peak of our heightened emotions, we could continue raging within our minds (maybe even coming up with all sorts of clever comebacks we wish we had said). However, after all the emotions calm down and you have a clear head and controlled emotions, perhaps you can be more objective.

Could it have been a discussion instead of an argument? Perhaps identifying the moment when the words turned spiteful is something you and your loved one can be more mindful of next time. Reflect on what you could have done differently and how to do that in the future. We can only control what we say and how we react. So, let's start there. But it takes a conscious effort, a dedication of time and energy to evaluate and identify opportunities for improvement. If we are constantly in a mode of charging ahead, we could be missing the mark when we finally arrive at our destination.

So, reflect often and don't wait until the end of your life to ponder: *I wish I had,* or *I wish I hadn't.* Don't live a life full of regrets. You can overcome regrets with reconciliation, and reconciliation starts with reflection.

OWNERSHIP IN HOW WE TURN OUT
TOMMY'S STORY

For a while, I was upset with my parents for not putting me in a better school when I was young. I believed that had I been in a better school, my future would have been brighter. My analytical, critical-thinking mind would have developed much better, my leadership skills significantly sharper. But instead, I went to a mediocre school and grew up exactly like that—mediocre.

This resentment bothered me more than I realized because when asked what I would tell my younger self if I had the chance, this bubbled to the top quickly. I wonder how much my underlying bitterness with my parents fueled our arguments as I was growing up. Had I expected more from them? Was I a lesser version of myself because of the poor choices they made?

As I pondered this more, I realized that yes, my parents decided to put me in that particular school, but it wasn't their *choice*. It was all they could afford—free education. Everything else was on me. It was *my* responsibility to get whatever I could out of my education. The Internet did not yet exist while I was a student, so there was no such thing as online information available at my fingertips; however, there were countless books in print I could have used to hone in on these skills I had deemed so important. True, as a student, I may not have had the maturity to realize exactly what skills would have served me better later in the working world. However, as a grown-up in the corporate world, it would have been on me to fill the gap.

It took deliberate reflection to come to this discovery. There was only so much I could blame on my parents. My expectation of them was misplaced and unfair. I had a much bigger part to play in my skillset and ongoing development.

ENABLING A BETTER FUTURE
JENNIFER'S STORY

My husband and I were fighting more frequently, usually about small things. But all our fights had two things in common: we always blew them out of proportion, and we weren't truly listening to each other.

By then, we were married for three years, and I realized that if we were to continue without any conscious effort for change, we would eventually live as co-habitants instead of spouses, hating each other—or divorced.

I knew something had to change, especially if we were going to have kids. We couldn't bring more lives into this world and expose them to a volatile home. However, it was hard to change alone. Improving a marriage requires both parties.

One day, I summoned up all my courage and blurted out, "I think we need marriage counseling."

Silence.

"I think we need marriage counseling," I repeated. "And if you don't want to join, that's okay, but I would like to start some sessions myself because I need to learn how to improve . . . *this*." I casually gestured to both of us.

After another pause, my husband finally said, "Okay. Let's go do it together."

I cannot describe the relief that washed over me right at that moment. Nothing had truly changed yet; we hadn't yet learned how to communicate better or have productive discussions.

But there was now *hope*.

Hope that the trajectory could change and offer a good chance at staying *happily* married. We had hope we could provide a loving home for our future children to witness real love upon which they would build their future family.

The counseling sessions were not always easy. But with each one, we were slowly moving away from the original doom and gloom path. With each session, we learned how to listen to and understand each other a little better. In the end, we learned to appreciate and love each other a whole lot more.

Reflection. Looking back so that the view looking forward is even clearer.

—Unknown

TAKEAWAYS

- Reflection isn't only about looking back and being bogged down with regrets; it can facilitate in identifying potential regrets in the future and enable a change of course in the present.

- Reflect often to stay on track toward your goals. If you find yourself failing to meet certain milestones, identify the culprits and try different ways to get back on track.

- Reflect backward and forward to see what areas you may want to allocate time for improvement.

9

MAXIMIZE YOUR SCHOOL YEARS

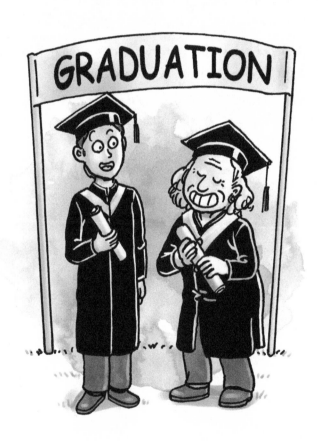

If you are not willing to learn no one can help you. If you are determined to learn no one can stop you.

—Zig Ziglar

I t is wise to strive for the highest possible level of education applicable to your life. Formal education is by no means the *only* avenue to making a good living, but it helps greatly to improve that chance. There are so many things you can learn to develop the skills needed to succeed in your career. Participating in projects with a range of personalities gives you a taste of navigating through real life by teaching you how to communicate and lead even those who don't want to be led.

Most people feel they wouldn't be able to do their job without a formal education. But following through with school isn't a guaranteed path to success. There are high school and college dropouts who became millionaires, but their path to success still took a lot of effort. Put in the work to understand what you enjoy.

Adjust when necessary. Don't feel like you need to stick with something just because you have already started down a certain path. But you owe it to yourself to make the most out of your education, not to only go through the motions so you can say you've graduated. If it's an option for you to finish school and pursue a higher level of education, go for it. You grow differently from graduate programs than undergraduate programs. No, they aren't for everyone and not a prerequisite for success. However, if you're chasing a career that values graduate degrees, then you'd be giving yourself a higher chance of success through your pursuit. Seek scholarships and financial grants if necessary; there is a lot of assistance available if you're willing to do your research. It can only help you.

People commonly regret they didn't take their education seriously. They prioritized partying and popularity over studying. In hindsight, it crushed them to know their family endured pain, worrying that high school graduation might not happen. So, don't throw away your precious school years succumbing to social pressures that may suggest academics aren't cool. There is nothing *uncool* about getting good grades. People who hold you back from doing well in school and judge you negatively when you are excelling aren't your true friends. Knowledge is a great asset that stays with you. Don't give it up for people who shouldn't matter and don't care enough about you. Make friends with those who would push you to try to do better in school, who can encourage you and hold you accountable. You can be well-liked and still do well in school.

A friend of mine was one of those authentically nice and smart guys in high school. People often called on him for help because he was reliable, down-to-earth, and compassionate. He was also extremely hard-working. While everyone else spent hours each day playing video games or hanging out at the mall, he was learning extensive computer programming beyond what the school taught. So, while the rest of us picked up part-time jobs paying minimum wage (back then, it was about $7 an hour), he was getting paid over $100 an hour doing programming for companies—as a high school student. Talk about a self-imposed, self-driven different trajectory. A single parent raised him who barely had time to spend with him, so he was by no means privileged. His accomplishments were due to his drive and focus. When he graduated from college, he was well-sought after by multiple big companies, making a six-figure salary right off the start.

Some people quit school early only to regret their decision later, typically when they are well into their careers and discover their lack of credentials were holding them back from advancement. Or they may notice they are the only one amongst their work peers to not have a certain degree or certification and feel they have fallen behind.

Others may have quit due to certain life circumstances, such as needing to start working early to support their family. What's great is to witness individuals who choose to go back to school to finish what they had started. There is no shame in finishing later. If anything, it's even more meaningful when you pursue your education because you truly appreciate its significance, not only because it's just the next thing to do in life.

DON'T LET STUBBORNNESS BLIND YOU
MY STORY

I avoided many subjects in high school that could have permitted me to truly understand what I'd enjoy and what I wouldn't. I was so sure I wanted to pursue a career in science that I very deliberately avoided all other subjects. To fulfill the minimum credit requirement of two courses in business, I chose *typing*. You read that right—*typing*.

My mom urged me on multiple occasions to at least try one business course. "Just try it to see if you'd like it. How could you be so sure you wouldn't like it?"

But somehow, I *knew*. I knew I loved learning biology and chemistry. I had an innate appreciation of nature and creation. The sheer anatomy of fruits and vegetables fascinated me. When I peeled an orange, I pondered the miraculous structure—how individual pulps form wedges, encased by an edible membrane, brought together to form an almost perfect sphere, further enveloped by a thick skin made up of different elements. And for every single orange to have the same uniformity to me was absolutely amazing. Don't even get me started on lettuce and cabbage and how each leaf overlaps the other so . . . gently. It's like they know how to grow and shape themselves before they even start sprouting.

And how our stomach knows how to digest all sorts of meat products but does not digest itself.

Yes, that's how mesmerized I was with science and nature and the amazing design behind all living things.

What I didn't consider was that I could also enjoy business, possibly even more so. I robbed myself of that chance. At least that's what happened in high school. One month after starting college, it dawned on me that I didn't know what to do with a science degree. I didn't want to become a doctor, nor did I want to spend my career in a lab. I enjoyed psychology, but over 1,500 psychology students in my Psychology 101 freshman class said the same thing. I explored a bit on what else I could do, and physical therapy intrigued me. My school was one of the few universities in Canada that offered this program, and they took seventy-five students each year out of tens of thousands of applicants. I suddenly realized I was no longer sure I wanted to pursue a career in science. I was afraid I'd be stuck with an occupation that chose me simply due to availability instead of the other way around.

I researched to see what it would take to switch to another faculty. It turned out that I had a shot at transferring over to Commerce, thankfully, because of my grades in my science courses.

Quickly, I fell in love with marketing and kept studying psychology on the side to satisfy that unceasing interest. I have been working in marketing-related jobs ever since.

I would urge my younger self to consider the possibility that she may have a higher interest in something she simply hasn't yet encountered. It does not have to *replace* science, but acknowledge that it's probable there is something else she would enjoy as a career even more. And what better time to explore than during school when it's practically free to do so (except for schools with tuitions), and you have more time and energy than you ever will the rest of your life.

THE DREAM TO SING FOR AN AUDIENCE
CATHERINE'S STORY

I wish I had joined a pop band. Secretly, I loved to sing, but because I told myself academics should come above extracurricular activities, I buried my nose in textbooks day and night. In turn, I removed the opportunity to develop an interest and a potential gift. I had a good voice and a wide range, but I wasn't a confident singer because I didn't have an outlet to practice. Other than singing when I was home alone, I couldn't convince myself to dedicate time and energy toward it, to make something of it, even if it was purely for fun. To me (and my parents), time spent studying was time well spent. And so that was my motto all through my school years. Had I pursued singing and learned to play pop music on the piano, I believe I would have grown up to be more well-rounded. My artistic and creative abilities would have developed more, which could have helped me with other areas of my life. Plus, my social circle would have grown. I wouldn't have hung out only with others who also chose to bury their noses in textbooks. My world would be so much broader.

PUSHING FOR MORE
VALERIE'S STORY

If I could choose all over again, I would have taken drama classes in high school. Why? Because it's the class that would have made me the *most uncomfortable*. And while in school, it's typical to fulfill the minimum credit requirements to graduate. But I had opted for the path of least resistance. And admittedly, there is enough to navigate and figure out in high school. Those are challenging years socially, physically, emotionally, and spiritually. But high school is a great opportunity to explore, discover your interests and talents, inside and outside of school. Drama classes could have propelled me further later in life. I wouldn't have such paralyzing stage fright that I'd completely blank out at the beginning of a piano recital despite practicing the same song every day for the past six months. I wouldn't be over ten years into my career and still terrified at the thought of presenting in front of a room full of people because I blush when all eyes are on me. And I wouldn't fail multiple commercial auditions with big-name brands because my acting was utterly *horrible*. I would have jumped at the chance of a friend offering to connect me to his agent for opportunities to be an extra on various TV series. No, it wasn't my desire to become a celebrity. But it would have been a fun, new experience had I had the ability to act well.

Looking back, I see now that I had created a very narrow arena for myself. Had I learned to face my discomfort early on, I would be more willing to step out of my comfort zone. I would not have lost anything by being more involved with drama. So what if I got a few laughs directed at me? I bet I wouldn't be the only novice in the class. To start at ground zero means I could only have improved. And even if they laughed at me, I think that would have helped thicken my skin to overcome bigger challenges in the future. Back in high school, the stakes seemed high. I was trying to avoid the potential humiliation. But in hindsight, the stakes have only grown as I aged. I could have found greater success at different points in my life had I learned to face my fear of being in front of an audience earlier on.

Learn as much as you can while you are young, since life becomes too busy later.

—Dana Stewart Scott

TAKEAWAYS

- Make the most out of your education. Don't give in to distractions. There is nothing uncool about doing well in school.

- Learn as much as you can while you are young, have more time, and your memory can still serve you well.

- Push yourself to learn something out of your comfort zone early on.

10

SELF-DISCIPLINE IS A GIFT

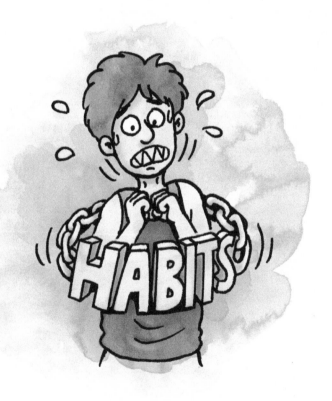

There is one thing that 99 percent of "failures" and "successful" folks have in common—they all hate doing the same things. The difference is successful people do them anyway.

—Darren Hardy

One of the best things you can do to set yourself up for an easier future is to learn self-discipline early on. Habits are hard to break, especially if you let them stick around for too long. By the same virtue, good habits can stay put and continue to serve you well when you practice them day in and day out. When you incorporate good habits into your life and allow them to become routine, you lay a positive foundation to uphold further good.

If you have bad posture, unless you intentionally and consciously correct it, your bad posture will continue, likely worsening over time. The same applies to your life. Be intentional about setting your path and getting rid of baggage and bad habits that hold you back. When you notice that it's not going the way you meant to go, lead the effort to reset. Don't leave it for someone else to do it for you. Remember, you're in the driver's seat.

BE GOOD TO YOUR BODY

It takes a lot of discipline to find time to work out, especially when juggling many other responsibilities such as keeping little ones fed and alive. For years I worked hard at being physically active—working out at the gym, weightlifting, running, etc. After the kids, all that came to a screeching halt. Life got insanely busy, and my husband and I operated on survival mode for a while. Who has time to work out when they have newborns and toddlers at home?

The lack of exercise gradually took a toll on my health. I got sick more often, my muscle mass became non-existent (made worse by aging), and I was tired all the time. It felt like I was wasting my physical health away.

Even though I still haven't *consistently* woven exercise back into my routine, I believe the first essential step is to recognize it's a lacking area and requires attention. It's a good thing our muscles have memory, but it has also been years since I truly worked out regularly. I hope my body can also forgive my prolonged neglect. As I fight against comfort and being too tired, even fifteen minutes of physical activity can counter the negativity. Once I committed to at least fifteen minutes of activity three times a week, I have found greater success at following it through.

I knew someone who was very envious of other guys with lean statures and six-pack abs (let's call him Jake.) He wasn't shy talking about how much he wished he had that stature, but he naturally was plumper than the average guy. Jake used to make fun of his potbelly. He understood his diet of processed carbs and high volumes of high-sugar snacks and beverages kept him from making the changes he desired. Since he had been this way as a kid, his diet needed a *major* makeover to start getting leaner, but it was one change he found extremely difficult to make.

Though I pass no judgment on his choices or physique, that's where discipline comes in. A fit, well-nourished body impacts many facets of our lives. And simply wishing for the perfect body does not yield results. It takes work—steady, consistent work, not binges, temporary diets, or random workouts. Developing healthful habits early on makes it easier to maintain a healthy body. When you establish the habit, it becomes maintenance instead of overhauling and resisting old habits.

So, be kind to your body early on. Protect it from toxins. Eat well, stay hydrated, and exercise.

REGULAR REST IS IMPORTANT TOO

Do yourself a favor and don't treat sleep like it's dispensable. Sleep is *extremely* important. When we are young, we tend to choose to stay up late at night and sleep in until noon. My dad used to get so frustrated with that behavior because half the day was over by the time I woke up. He thought it was the biggest waste of time (and sunlight!). But our bodies have an internal clock where we need to rest by a certain time for optimal repairing and rejuvenating. You may not notice the effects of sleep deprivation because our bodies tend to be quite forgiving and resilient when we are young. But it catches up. Some people speak of premature wrinkles and veins on their eyelids from staying up late chronically and having way too much screen time.

I certainly saw how much my face aged in the few seasons of my life when sleep did become a luxury. First, when I worked full-time while pursuing my master's degree on an accelerated, part-time basis, I slept no more than four hours on most days that year. The next two were when my children were born. I expected to look tired, but looking back at those photos is utterly heartbreaking. I must have aged more than five years in one. With my second child, the effect of severe sleep deprivation was even more destructive. I believe it was simply because I was older, and my body was less able to bounce back.

Don't get me wrong; I am not arguing that aging is bad. We are all aging every day. But there is a reason your body and mind need quality rest. Sleep isn't non-purposeful; sleep is good. And it certainly is *not* a guilty pleasure. Downtime is critical for your body and brain to revitalize and recharge.

BATTLING AGAINST TEMPTATIONS

Life comes with a lot of temptations. And they seem to increase as time goes on. One temptation that seems to affect a lot of people nowadays is to spend time on unproductive and unvaluable things. It has become a challenge to stay focused and not give in to distractions.

When we are in the middle of doing our work, how often do we check our phones for messages, the latest news, or our friends' photos? If we counted the number of times we get distracted by a phone notification, we may be astonished by how disruptive our work pattern is. Sometimes, even when our phone isn't alerting us of an incoming message or update, we may find ourselves still reaching for the screen to see what the latest social media posts are. In other words, even when we aren't prompted, we are still proactively reaching out to the distraction.

Don't we all know someone who cannot put their phone down for more than a minute? At a work meeting, a colleague continually checked his phone at least every ten seconds. He unlocked his phone, checked for notifications, and shut the screen off, only to repeat again a few seconds later. This is detrimental behavior for a work environment as it is impossible to properly grasp what others are saying.

When we have a negative habit leading us down the wrong path, it's important to address it. That means our action and response need to guide us back to the path that gets us to where we want to be. If you are easily distracted by your phone and wish to reduce the time you spend mindlessly scrolling through social media, you can try one of these options:

- Deactivate or uninstall all the apps that are at the root of the distractions—this is the most extreme approach. Going cold turkey is sometimes what some people need to make a clean break from something they know is hurting them.

- Do a fast, such as not going on any social media for a month—this is another form of going cold turkey, but there is an end date. This could work in your favor as the cut-off may not seem as permanent, but it can also work against you if you resume the old habit at the end of the month.

- Limit the time spent on social media to, say, no more than thirty minutes per day. This may require external support like an accountability partner, or you could set your phone to block your usage once you have reached your thirty-minute mark. The key is not to allow yourself to slide where thirty minutes can become forty minutes and so on.

- Put your phone away when you need to focus on your work, so that you are not distracted by notifications. Set your phone to only allow emergency calls to come through. The more you get used to the lack of notifications, the easier it will become to not constantly reach for your phone.

- Take a step back to assess your VIPs, then find other methods to stay in touch. So much of social media is completely irrelevant and does not contribute to our development or relationships. The more we pay attention to those time-sucking posts, the more these apps target us with similar information, presenting more noise for us to ignore.

MORE ON SELF-DISCIPLINE

There are other ways self-discipline can help with your success and well-being:

- **Read.** Absorb as much as you can while you're young and your brain can still easily retain new information and knowledge, especially when you aren't raising a family. When you have a young kid, free time is scarcer. So be disciplined about reading books that feed your mind and expand your thinking. Books are wonderful teachers.

- **Don't Skip Class.** When we are young, our teachers discipline us in school as do our parents at home. Entering college can be a rude awakening for a lot of people. Suddenly, no one checks to be sure you attend classes, complete your readings, submit your assignments. It is all up to you. Even for those who are studious and enjoy school, there may be days when you have to fight the urge to skip class. Professors hold classes for a reason, so even if you think you can skip and catch up, it is almost certainly best to attend.

- **Wear sunscreen.** I have heard countless people approaching their late thirties or early forties say they regret how they subjected their skin to sun abuse while they were young. Sunspots eventually show up as a nagging reminder, and they tend to get darker and more prominent over time. In some instances, the first warning sign of sun overexposure may even be skin cancer.

- **Don't procrastinate.** If you can do it today, then don't leave things for tomorrow. Yes, every day has priorities, but don't practice laziness. If it's important, tackle it now. Our tasks and accomplishments build upon each other. Procrastination today leads to the delay of tomorrow's productivity. Remember, you reap what you sow. When an important paper is worth 50% of your college course grade, it would be unwise to wait to begin it the night before it's due. Believe me, I'm speaking from experience. Even if you pull an all-nighter with the best of intentions, the result will be a rush job, lacking substance and depth. And, in my case, the grade matched the effort. It was not my finest work nor something I was proud of.

- **Manage your reactions.** Very few people can control their emotions 100% of the time. Raw reactions can lead us to trouble and to say things we don't truly mean. Losing your cool in a work setting can come across as unprofessional and might even cause career-limiting damage. Once, I observed a man slam his fist on the table in a meeting, dropped an F-bomb, and stormed out of the conference room in frustration. From the expression on everyone's face, it was obvious people considered the reaction inappropriate, especially in the workplace. Regardless of his reasoning or if others agreed with the frustration, the rude reaction was uncalled for. Would you prefer to have a calm and collected leader or one who has a hot temper? I'm guessing most of you (or perhaps all of you) would say the former. It is difficult to work for someone who is a ticking time bomb. It'd be like walking on eggshells at all times. And with that, apply it to how you may want to discipline your temperament. This is not a suggestion to snuff out your anger; we all have a right to feel angry. But how we choose to display that anger and treat others is a different matter altogether. Anger and frustration are not reasons for disrespect nor contempt. Your actions speak more about your character.

- **Seek feedback regularly and use it to continue improving.** Don't let discomfort with hearing feedback stop you. You could be holding yourself back from making a profound change that could lead to a much better future for yourself and those you care about.

- **Invest in acts of kindness regularly.** Every time you help someone—even in a small way—blesses others. There are countless ways to help others: a simple word of encouragement, paying for someone's meal, calling a friend to see how they're doing, praying for someone, extending financial assistance to someone in need, lending a hand with a D.I.Y. project, helping a new mother so she can get some quality rest, delivering meals to the senior community—the possibilities are endless. It's a blessing to give rather than to receive. And it is good for your soul.

NIP IT IN THE BUD
ROSIE'S STORY

I had just moved to a new city and a new school. As a newcomer, everything was an adjustment. I was a bit on the shy side, so it was hard for me to make new friends. Therefore, I spent a lot of time communicating with my friends back home. Soon, this took a toll on my study time after school, especially when my friends were several hours ahead of me because of our time difference. I constantly chatted with them for hours each day via instant messaging, texting, and social media. It helped me feel connected and tamed my homesickness, but it was increasingly challenging to keep up with school. I knew I needed intervention.

When I confided in my father about my struggles, he did not scold me and gave me credit for acknowledging that I needed help. He advised that I delete all the communication apps, rationalizing that if it was that difficult for me to stop myself from getting on the apps, the best thing was to get rid of the root of the temptation, which was the access to the apps.

He explained it's like the struggle with a gambling addiction; not stepping foot inside a casino would be easier than being there and fighting the temptation.

I had to nip it in the bud.

It was a painful process. It felt like cutting off all the friendships I was trying so hard to maintain while not having new friends to fill the void. However, I knew it was necessary and saw that continuing the current behavior would lead me to fail my courses.

I am glad I found the courage to ask my dad for help. He told me what I *needed* to hear, not what I *wanted* to hear. He didn't give me the easy way out. I am thankful he had the confidence in me to do the right thing.

BE DISCIPLINED ABOUT MATERIAL THINGS
MICHELLE'S STORY

I grew up without clutter in the home. We lived by this rule: for every newly purchased item, we had to find an old one to give away. This ensured manageable volumes in toy bins, drawers, and closets. I hated this rule as a child. Wanting a new toy didn't mean I liked my existing ones any less, yet this one-in-one-out policy meant just that.

When I grew older and shared living spaces with others, I appreciated this habit. I couldn't assume space was unlimited. It also helped me financially. To buy something new, I had to make sure I *really* wanted it, not just because it was on sale. Otherwise, I'd risk having to throw away something I adored.

For God has not given us a spirit of fear and timidity, but of power, love, and self-discipline.

—2 Timothy 1:7

TAKEAWAYS

- Learn to self-discipline early on so it becomes something you naturally do. It'd help you stay on track as you progress toward your goals.

- Be ruthless with bad habits. Cut it off as soon as you can. Seek help and support if needed. Don't keep bad habits around out of comfort.

- Be disciplined with your health, your development, and how you treat people.

11

MASTER YOUR FINANCES

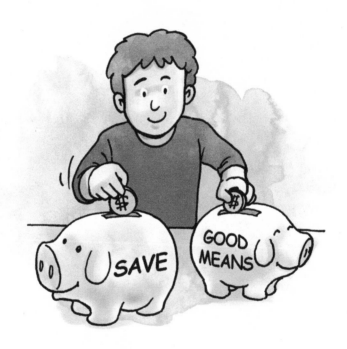

You must gain control over your money or the lack of it will forever control you.

—Dave Ramsey

One of the most important things to learn as soon as possible is how to manage your finances properly. If you grasp the foundations early on, you can avoid a lot of stress for yourself and your loved ones in the future. One should not underestimate financial stress. Finances are said to be one of the major causes of divorce.[1] Something this powerful can work in your favor if you learn to master it early.

The best part is, it's possible. It's possible to take control before it takes over your life. It's possible to not let it be a wedge in your family. It's possible to not let it be damaging to your well-being.

MONEY TALK DOESN'T HAVE TO BE SCARY

Here is the thing about money. It can be very basic and easy to understand. Though it can get more complicated if you want to get into it, it doesn't need to be.

---

[1]   Meyers, S. (2012, December 6). *How Financial Problems & Stress Cause Divorce.* Psychology Today. https://www.psychologytoday.com/us/blog/insight-is-2020/201212/how-financial-problems-stress-cause-divorce

If you are intimated by financial management, first learn to think of it in simple terms. Find people who are wise with money and good at teaching and see if they can give you a crash course. Sometimes, it only takes someone to explain a topic in a simplistic manner that gives you that *ah-ha* moment.

There are also a lot of free resources you can leverage to get a handle on key concepts as it comes to managing your money. Look for trustworthy sources online and start reading articles to try to improve your understanding.

Don't let it intimidate you. Don't give it more power than it should have. Money isn't a bad thing. It's a necessary part of our lives. Learn how to integrate it effectively into your life and goals.

And don't procrastinate. The longer you delay, the more you allow it to run unleashed in your life, which could be disastrous in the long run. Know that it's okay to take baby steps but keep pushing yourself to learn a little at a time. Then, put it into practice and keep practicing, and you'll soon realize your fear may have stemmed from a sense of unfamiliarity—we tend to be uncomfortable with unfamiliar things. So, get familiar. Find a friend to learn with. Whatever may help put you at ease, give it a try. And if it doesn't work, try something else. Don't let up. Money management is a part of our lives whether we like it or not. Either we control money, or it controls us. So, why not turn it into a friend and learn to work with it. Your future you will thank you for it.

LIVE WITHIN YOUR MEANS

Don't spend more than you make. It's very simple but so critical. If you spend more than you make, you will run out of money. Yes, credit cards could tide you over, but the point is not to buy things on credit, *especially if you cannot pay off your credit card balance in full when it's due.* I understand circumstances and situations arise sometimes, and I'm not judging that. But don't set out allowing yourself to get into this spending habit. It leads nowhere and only digs a bigger hole. The bigger the hole, the harder it is to get out of it. $500 may not seem like a big balance right now, but it can quickly snowball to $5,000 or more. $5,000 can be a daunting sum to pay off if you are barely making ends meet today. With high interest rates, $5,000 could quickly multiply before you know it. Don't tell yourself: *I'll pay it off in the future.* Where you can help it, don't set your future up to be paying for your past. Your future will come with its own financial responsibilities. Do what you can now to alleviate the future burden instead of adding to it.

Some people who have a hard time living within their means often find their success comes from cutting up their credit cards. This eliminates the temptation to spend on credit. It also eliminates the stress of mounting debt in the background. And if it seems like a light matter and you find yourself dealing with a growing amount of debt, perhaps it's your perception of it that's doing you a disservice. Perhaps if your mindset were to shift to seeing debt as a foe, something to eliminate instead of to embrace, you may not be so comfortable letting it accumulate.

Living frugally is a good habit to adopt. The idea of being frugal with yourself seems to scare a lot of people. Perhaps it's because when people hear frugal, they think cheap. They think it means to deprive themselves *severely* of the joys of life. But if you look at the definition of frugal, it's to use money more wisely, to prioritize your spending. Frugal means to be diligent with your resources. It means not to waste. Let's face it, when we take a hard look at where our money goes, we can likely identify some areas where we could put it to better use.

As you earn more, you may find yourself tempted to take on a more lavish lifestyle. It's important to make sure your new expenses don't surpass your increased income. The more you can keep your expenses at a similar level, the more you have left to save for your future.

LEARN HOW TO SAVE

When you are young—especially if you're single—saving is more important. It's a time when you can make a lot of decisions without it impacting anyone else significantly. When you have a family, your financial decisions affect more than just you. And when you have a family, your expenses may be exponentials of what they are when you are single and unattached. This is a time to make wise choices. Learn to build a habit of discerning between must-haves versus nice-to-haves. *Must-haves* are things like electricity, transportation, housing (like rent or mortgage), meals (basic, yet nutritious); *nice-to-haves* are things that aren't critical for your day-to-day like fancier clothes, a pantry full of snacks, and entertainment. Sure, allow yourself to indulge once in a while, but it doesn't have to be daily. A friend of mine spent $5 to $10 on coffee and breakfast every morning, then at least another $10 on lunch, oftentimes more. One day, as she was trying to find areas to cut down her expenses, she realized she was easily spending $15–$20 every day. Over thirty days, that's $450–$600 on breakfast and lunch! When she layered on going out to dinner and attending social gatherings, she discovered she spent over $1,000 each month on meals. By making coffee at home and preparing her breakfast and lunch for at least half the month, she cut this budget down by almost half. So, she was able to save about $500 each month from her previous routine and still enjoyed splurging on coffee, breakfast, lunch, and dinner two weeks out of a month. $500 a month equates to $6,000 a year. How would you be able to make use of an extra $6,000 a year simply from changing a small habit?

Learn to save aggressively for your retirement and your children's education. Every year you postpone your savings, you're losing the compounding effect, practically robbing yourself of more dollars from your retirement and future enjoyments and possibly robbing your children of a better education. There is also the option just to retire later, but it might not be entirely your choice. Your skillset will need to be relevant; the job market will need to be open and in a good state; your health and energy level will need to sustain you.

Saving early also builds you a safety net for later if life throws you a curveball, you want a career change, go back to school, or start a business. Sometimes, these things don't allow you to maintain a full-time job. And sometimes, it makes more sense to devote all your time to your new endeavor. Wouldn't it be nice to have the flexibility to go back to school full-time so you can truly concentrate while you still have money to cover your basic needs? Or, if you have a financial cushion, you can pursue a dream venture without worrying about your daily expenses. Building that safety net gives you options. Even if you don't need it, it doesn't hurt to have it available. Taking financial burdens out of the equation as you evaluate options for your career can make a world of difference. I know people who saved up enough to go back to school full-time to support a complete career change, to pay for their master's degree to facilitate career advancement, to go abroad and volunteer for two years, to quit their steady job to become an entrepreneur, and to take a break from a mundane job. These are not easy moves. It takes courage and faith. It certainly helps if financial provisions are not a major obstacle.

Here are some tips on saving money that have helped other individuals:

- For every dollar you spend on something that isn't necessary, set aside the same amount in savings. If it's a bigger ticketed item, allow yourself to save that same amount over time. The key is to land the same amount in savings as you put out in spending.

- For every new pair of shoes you buy, you have to throw out an old pair. This would make sure you only buy what you truly love and will cherish. This tip has allowed significant money savings because it helps to cut down impulsive shopping. Don't buy something you *somewhat like* because it's on sale. Typically, these are things you only wear once before you abandon them. Or worse yet, they hang in the closet with the tag still on. If it's not worth giving up something you already own and love, it's not worth wasting your money on.

- When building a budget, put something in the "save" bucket first. Make that your most protected chunk that comes out of your paycheck.

- Stick with sales for things as much as possible— clothes, shoes, necessities, groceries. Saving $10 or $20 here and there can amount to quite a significant sum over time.

PUT YOUR MONEY TO GOOD USE

I believe it is important to invest in your future and your children's future. And with that, turn the cash you have today into more money for tomorrow. Put your money to work. It's only depreciating in value if you keep it under your mattress, in a jar, or barely earning a penny in interest in your bank account.

Yes, the money market has its ups and downs. If you are risk-averse, choose low-risk options that could still give you a healthy return by the time you need the money, like when you retire. Find a good financial advisor and leverage their expertise. Not knowing *how* is not good enough of a reason not to do something with your money.

Take your retirement financial needs seriously and be responsible about them. When we are young, retirement may seem like a century away. However, while we are young is when we should take advantage of this extended time frame and set ourselves up for a financially stable retirement. When we are twenty, something we put aside has so much more potential to accumulate to a good sum when we retire at sixty-five than if we were to set it aside when we are forty. The former would have given us an extra twenty years (*two decades!*) for the money to grow. Let's say you invest $100 every month beginning when you are twenty years old. At an average annual return rate of 10% (i.e., on average, every year the money you have in the investment grows by 10%), you would end up with over $1,050,000 by the time you reach sixty-five years of age. A friend who starts setting aside the same $100 per month when they are forty years old will have just over $133,000 when they reach sixty-five years of age. You will have invested a total of $54,000, spread out over forty-five years. Your friend will have invested $30,000, spread out over twenty-five years. But your $54,000 can turn into over a million dollars, likely allowing you a decent retirement, especially if you let your investment continue generating a return, even if you were to cease your monthly contribution of $100 after sixty-five.

Don't bank on an inheritance to tide you over at retirement. Work for your retirement. And by the same token, don't plan on having your children take care of you financially when you retire. They will have their *own* burdens to bear. If they can support you financially throughout your retirement, consider that a blessing. But don't depend on it; free them of that responsibility. It's one of the best gifts you can give them. And relying on them may be too much of a gamble for your own good. If this doesn't pan out, you would have very few options.

Some of you might be born into situations where money is in abundance, and you don't need to worry. Or perhaps you are doing so well in your career that there is no need to stick to a tight budget. If that's you, may I encourage you to be more generous with your financial means? $40 might be a meal (or perhaps a portion of one), but $40 could sponsor a child in an undeveloped country for a whole month. That same $40 could pay for the food, clean water, education, school supplies, and medical care for a child in need. So even if you have more money than you know what to do with, there are still good reasons to be frugal.

The money you consider loose change may be what someone needs for survival.

Everyone can experience the joy and blessing of generosity; because everyone has something to give.

—Jan Grace

IT'S POSSIBLE TO MASTER YOUR FINANCES
SCOTT'S STORY

To this day, I still recall noticing something different—special—about one of the trainees who showed up in my corporate classroom one Monday morning some years ago.

He carried this level of confidence that was unusual for his age. Just starting in his career, he had recently completed his college degree.

Over time, I appreciated his sense of curiosity and inquisitive mind more and more. He asked excellent questions, never quite coming across as being insecure for not knowing the answer.

During the multi-week training, I learned of his financial acumen. Even though he did not have a finance degree, he spoke like he had his finances figured out—like he had already, despite his young age, mastered his finances. He was a dedicated saver, but he also understood when and where to invest his money. I was pretty sure he already had a good stash set aside toward his retirement.

One day, I couldn't hold back anymore. I had to ask.

"How did you learn to be so good with money?"

"I am the youngest in the family with three older brothers. I have observed them since I was young, watching their choices and results. Our family wasn't well off. We had to live with tight budgets, but we also learned to make the most out of what we had. My brothers handled every dollar with purpose; they were responsible for what each dollar could mean *in the future*, not only looking for ways to spend it today for instant gratification. I asked them a lot of questions and tried my best to learn from them. And I *still* ask a lot of questions. And they always take the time to share their insights and knowledge with me. But I always have to ask. They aren't sitting around waiting to give me financial crash courses. If I want to learn, it's on me to take that initiative."

I was envious of this young man and the natural opportunity he was born into. Not everyone has families with such financial attentiveness and rigor, I certainly don't. However, that doesn't mean help isn't available. It means we have to look elsewhere. We need to be responsible for our financial knowledge and proactive in mastering our money. Meeting this young man was a great reminder to myself that the ability to master our finances exists. The ownership and accountability lie with us.

Financial literacy is just as important in life as the other basics.

—John W. Rogers Jr.

TAKEAWAYS

- Gain better financial knowledge as early as you can. Don't let it intimidate you. Seek help from other financially wise people.

- Live within your means and prioritize saving over spending on nice-to-haves.

- Be generous with your money. And the more you manage your finances well, the more you can help others.

12

ENRICH YOUR SOCIAL NETWORK

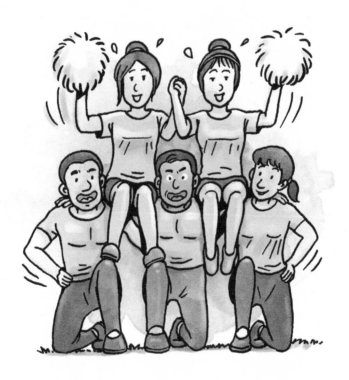

We find our humanity—our will to live and our ability to love—in our connections to one another.

—Sheryl Sandberg

Humans need interaction. In this day and age, technology allows for self-entertainment without connection to others. It's more possible than ever to live like a hermit and not feel bored. You may feel lonely, but there are endless ways to use your time alone. We connect through our phones *when we want to*. We respond *when we want to*. We can pretend to be busy even if we are not. We display a version of ourselves for others to see that may or may not be the truth.

Some people love their alone time. Most people *need* time to themselves. Solitude can be great for the mind, heart, and soul. It can be a time of recuperation and renewal and a time to rid yourself of external pressures and slow down and breathe.

However, enjoying alone time doesn't require walls and shields away from the rest of the world. We need connections. It's how we were made—to be a part of a bigger whole. It's critical to feel a part of something without judgment, to feel supported when in need, and to feel encouraged to do and be better.

Sometimes, these connections forge naturally as we transition through different life stages. When I first moved to Hawai'i for a new job, I barely knew anyone. A lot of my colleagues reached out and offered their support and genuine care, which ultimately made my move thousands of miles away from home much easier. They looked out for me. They took me surfing (or at least what was my attempt at it) and hiking on weekends to help me acclimate. They kept me up to date on social events so I could go out and experience the local lifestyle. Left on my own, I might have opted to stay in my comfort zone.

My colleagues also kept a close eye on me when we had a serious tsunami threat, hung out with me outside of the office, worked out with me after work so I wouldn't have to run alone and to be sure I was safe. They invited me along to holiday gatherings knowing I'd be home alone otherwise and were, in my eyes, *my family*.

When I became a mom for the first time, I had an amazing outpouring of support from other mothers who understood what I was going through. There was also an outpouring of support from other non-mom friends who wanted to celebrate with me. They all showered me with an abundance of gifts, an amazing diaper cake (makes sense that they call it a baby shower!), many words of wisdom to help prepare me, and empathy for the challenges I would face as a new mother. But it was truly the love behind everything that touched my heart the most.

Sometimes connections can take some effort. You may find yourself lost in a big crowd at a school, a church, an organization, or a community. It's easy to hide in the shadows and go unnoticed. But over time, you may find your sense of belonging declining or outright lacking as though everyone is together on a shared mission and you're just . . . *there*. You may feel a lack of meaningful engagement. There may be certain seasons when you need to focus on whatever else is going on in your life and minimize extracurricular activities. But when you are able, invest in connecting with people and building relationships. These could very well become your lifeline in a time of need. Or you could be that very lifeline that could make a significant difference in someone else's life.

For some, the initial outreach to make connections is nerve-racking. Not everyone is a people person. However, sometimes putting yourself in a setting with others opens up the door for friendships. Sometimes one small step helps us connect, perhaps to someone we will need before realizing we need them.

WHO DO YOU SURROUND YOURSELF WITH?

Typically, we tend to stick with people and things familiar to us. Birds of a feather flock together. Like attracts like, so the saying goes. We tend to talk and think like those we hang out with the most. Sometimes we may even find we dress alike.

I still recall when a new friend of my best friend met me for the first time. He said to her, "Now it makes so much sense why you dress the way you do." I guess we dressed alike but never noticed it!

So, we can also groom ourselves to be a better version of ourselves by who we spend our time with. It helps to surround ourselves with grounded, loyal people, those who can guide us back on the right path when we veer off. People who are willing to invest time in you, your life, your well-being, for *your good*, not theirs. Friends who will truly stick by you through thick and thin. These people are disciplined, genuinely care, want you to be successful, and don't see your success as a threat to their worth. These people have good, solid relationships in their lives and want you to do well. They are inspirational.

These types of friends are rare. And as we mature, it could become harder to establish solid friendships. If you find someone like that later in life, consider yourself very blessed.

When you are with good people, you lift each other. Iron sharpens iron, as they say.

But if we get involved with the wrong people who have bad intentions and don't truly care about our well-being, things can easily go the other way. You could spiral downward. And when you find yourself fighting alone, it's hard to change course and spiral back up. You will need strong, good people to help you do that. It's not impossible to do it on your own, but it certainly would be easier if you have people to lean on through the rough patches.

Think about the people who are in your close circle. What are they like? Are they a positive influence on you? Do they inspire you to grow? Do they help you thrive? If you were to be like them, would you be content?

You are the average of the five people you spend the most time with.

—Jim Rohn

DIVERSITY MATTERS

While we can learn from one best friend or a few great friends, we can also learn from others. Having friends from all walks of life could expose us to new things we wouldn't encounter otherwise. There could be something very specific you learn from each friend and together, that can shape you like no one person can.

I have good friends who are old enough to be my parents, and I cherish these friendships tremendously. These people have shared their wisdom and life experiences; I always learn something from our chats. They are amazing individuals to begin with and even more so for pouring into my life and considering me as a peer, an equal. Through this, they have shown me the manifestation of true humility. And I have come to realize that it's truly down to what you choose to do with what you learn from your friends. You can take the *good-for-them* attitude and leave it as such. Or you can get more out of it by being thoughtful about what they are sharing with you and how you may be able to apply it to your life and build upon it.

It's also important to connect with people who are different from us. It's natural for us to associate with those just like us—in appearance, ethnicity, language, values, and faith.

We were all made to be different; that's part of the beauty of the human race. Unfortunately, we are often uncomfortable in embracing differences. Somehow, we may feel insecure and awkward when we hang with others unlike us.

If you find yourself feeling this way, bear in mind that differences aren't necessarily bad. And similarities aren't always good. Differences can help us see things we never tried before, expand our horizons, and complement our weaknesses.

Don't assume that just because someone is different, that their way is inferior. It's just that—*different.*

And if we can't quite grasp their perspectives or means, keep an open mind that perhaps it's because we can't comprehend, not because our ways are better.

140

Approach differences with curiosity, and it can be quite a fun adventure to see a whole new world, or, for some, it can be daunting, for it goes against what we instinctively do. Immigrants arriving in a new country tend to seek out people from their hometown and gel together. And it makes sense. Being with people from the same background gives a sense of familiarity, making a move to a foreign country less terrifying. Add the possibility of not speaking the new language, and it supports why people may choose not to break out of their social bubbles. It's safe. It's comforting. It lends support. But as you enter a new place, there are so many new things to learn. The opportunities are endless! Learn the new cuisine, understand pop culture, local slang, what people celebrate. Push yourself a little to get engaged and blend in. It doesn't make you lose your sense of self or where you originated. It merely opens your eyes up to other parts of this beautiful place we call Earth.

MAKE IT A TWO-WAY STREET

Having an enriched social network does not mean you are only taking from others. Meaningful and authentic friendships take bidirectional love, respect, and effort. Make an effort to reach out and connect. It could be a quick check-in with a good friend once a week or, as life gets busier, perhaps even once a month. It's good for your well-being and your friend's. Don't sit and wait for people to come to you. If everyone waited for someone else to reach out first, friendships would evaporate.

We were made for connection, to lift others. Be a source of love and encouragement. You may have no idea how much a friend needs that right now.

SEEING THE WORLD WITH NEW EYES
MICHAEL'S STORY

I am a single child, which comes with many implications in life, like playing by myself a lot. Truthfully, I can't remember if I enjoyed it or if I simply grew to accept it as a way of life.

In my teenage years, I had many opportunities to travel. Perhaps it helped that my family enjoyed seeing the world. I soon shared their love for being out there and experiencing new things.

Even in my hometown, I have come to realize I don't have just one circle of friends, one clique, so to speak. I hang out with many different circles of friends. Sometimes, I do get this sense that I don't belong to a particular group, like I don't have a home base. But then, I think of all the different groups of friends who cherish my friendship, and I realize I am truly blessed. Perhaps being a single child equipped me to be comfortable being alone and also taught me how I can weave my way through different social settings.

I have also come to realize that I have learned so much from the diversity of my friends. There is something so fascinating about every culture in the world, and it's through these friendships I've been afforded the opportunity to understand their traditions, cuisines, and language. People appreciate your genuine interest in understanding their culture. And the more I learn, the more I want to understand. My friends enjoy taking me to restaurants that serve their cuisine so they can introduce me to new dishes. It's a fun learning experience for me, and they love to have someone to share their customs with.

My current job requires quite a bit of traveling. And I try to get the most out of each trip, no matter how rushed. I push myself to go out there to experience something new and meet new people. People can teach you so much, especially when they are quite different from you. I am often baffled by people who only want to stick with those who are just like them; what's the fun in that? And what's there to learn?

I have grown so much from observing and conversing with people of different backgrounds. Hearing their stories alone make me never want to say goodbye. And I can honestly say my eyes are now more open than ever, and I never want to stop learning more.

> *If only you could sense how important you are to the lives of those you meet; how important you can be to people you may never even dream of. There is something of yourself that you leave at every meeting with another person.*
>
> —Fred Rogers

TAKEAWAYS

- Build connections and a strong support network.

- Surround yourself with good people. We tend to become more like those with whom we spend our time.

- Diversity matters. Expand your social circle with people who are different from you; it'd open your eyes to so much more of what this world has to offer.

13

MENTORS ARE ANGELS
IN DISGUISE

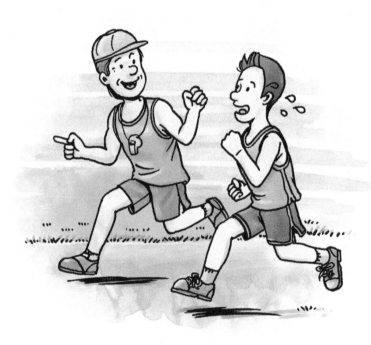

If you ask any successful business person, they will always have had a great mentor at some point along the road.

—Richard Branson

One of the best things you can do to help yourself propel forward, reach your goals faster, and get better at what you do is to have mentors. Mentors can offer wisdom on different aspects of your life such as careers, relationships, and parenting, so it's important to have multiple mentors. Much like you have different teachers and coaches to teach you different subjects and extracurricular activities while you were in school, mentors can guide on different facets of life to help you grow and learn.

Like a sports coach, a mentor can be area-specific to help you improve, because no matter how good we are at something, we can still get better. A mentor in your industry can guide you along the way up the corporate ladder as far as you desire. If you are trying to figure out what career to major in, a mentor in your field(s) of interest can help add clarity, guide you through the decisions, and discover things you may otherwise not know. For example, if you are considering becoming a doctor but are not positive you want to do that for the rest of your life, it'd help to conduct more research first. Medical school is a huge investment of time and money! If you know you want to become a doctor but feel uncertain what specialty to choose, take some time to talk to different doctors instead of leaping blindly and risking it not being what you want to do. Take the time to understand their day-to-day activities and the joys and struggles with their jobs. All jobs have pros and cons, so learn what they are up front to embark with the right expectations.

It is hard to speculate whether we'd enjoy certain careers in broad strokes; speaking to people who have experience could paint a more realistic picture.

MENTORS CAN HELP IN SO MANY WAYS

Mentors are great at helping with soft skills. Want to improve your leadership skills? Communications skills? That is where mentors and coaches can really make an impact. No matter how good you may already be at speaking in front of people, a remarkable communicator can help you further polish your performance. Likewise, leadership is more of an art than a science. Many corporate executives still require coaching, even if they are already effective in what they do. I have heard a lot of executives make references to their mentors, which highlights an ongoing need for mentorship.

If you can think of some stand-out leaders in your life, reach out to them to see if they can mentor you, especially if this is an area you wish to refine. You do not need to aim to lead large corporations; good leadership skills can benefit you in many elements of life. Seek especially those who are servant leaders. From my observation, true servant leadership has the biggest following. They lead to help others be better and invest in others selflessly and not as part of boosting their own reputation or success.

Another area you might want to consider finding mentors are for the relationships in your life. If you are married or engaged, marital mentors could greatly help. Marriages are rarely free from conflict. We can even have conflicts with *ourselves*. Suddenly, building a life with someone we (typically) haven't known for that long, with whom we have clear differences and may not always agree with—someone we need to put before ourselves—is a tough thing to do *consistently*. It is hard to wake up every day with a mindset to serve and to love unconditionally.

It may be a honeymoon period for some with rosy days and not too many demands during the first year of marriage. But as time goes on, it is not uncommon to grow tired. Sometimes, our moods and stress from other areas take over, and we grow weary. Our spouse's flaws begin to irritate us. Sometimes, it's the traits we were attracted to in the beginning that end up being annoyances! But marital mentors with strong marriages themselves (usually not by luck but through hard work, dedication, and selflessness) can show us how to positively grow our marriage, overcome tough times, and love the other person even when they may not be easy to love.

This extends to when you have children in the picture, which greatly changes the dynamics in the household. A couple with a solid marriage could transfer their relational skills to effective parenting strategies and techniques. They would want to look for ways to continue evolving and improving their parenting methods, trying to see what works with their kids, catering to their uniqueness. People who have been through this have a lot of insights and wisdom to offer. Their experiences may differ from yours, but they likely would have suggestions for things you may want to try. They may also have insights into what pitfalls to avoid and help encourage you through parenting tribulations.

Keep in mind that mentorship can take various forms. It can be very official where you regularly meet weekly, biweekly, monthly, or quarterly. Those typically have a path or a curriculum as part of the mentorship with defined goals and milestones. Others can be more informal where you meet as needed. Sometimes, it can be for a particular season in your life, such as when trying to build on a venture or transitioning between jobs. It can get even more casual where you do not officially label it as a mentorship but engage in learning topic-specific discussions, like the example at the beginning of this chapter on learning about various medical specialties. These types are still knowledge-filled, but it's not quite like a mentor-mentee relationship.

There is one more effective form of mentorship often overlooked—reading books. With the countless books out there, there is a ton of knowledge readily available for your consumption. It's up to you when and how you expose yourself to the information and apply it to your life. So, if you can't think of anyone you could approach right now as a mentor, start by exploring books. They can open your eyes like never before.

FINDING A MENTOR

When looking for a mentor, find someone you respect and admire, someone who has established and achieved what you want to learn and adopt. If they seem out of your league, do not speak on their behalf and think they would reject your request before you even ask. That would only rob you of opportunities to grow. Mentorships are important enough to put yourself out there. Go and ask. The worst-case scenario is they say no. People who are good at what they do are understandably busy and may face many demands on their time and skillset. Do not let that keep you from taking initiative. If they cannot accept a mentee at this time, you can still ask if a one-off meeting is possible. If not, they may have someone else to recommend. Or maybe they will suggest you reach out again at a later time. If everyone shied away from approaching these strong potentials, they would not have any mentees. So, do yourself a favor and ask. Many people naturally want to help others and try to find the time to do so.

Be prepared with your list of questions or topics you'd like to discuss when you attend your mentorship session, especially at the beginning when establishing the relationship. A mentorship is not a setting where the mentee waits for downloadable information. The mentee has a responsibility to ensure the sessions and relationship are meaningful and productive. So, go with specific questions. Things can progress from there, and the mentor may have ideas on how to structure subsequent meetings, but please, take this very seriously. Someone is investing their time and energy to help you without expecting something in return.

I have various mentors in my life, and I am grateful for each of them. They have all greatly enriched my life, poured into me, and helped to renew my heart and soul. Even when I may not have specific problems, they have a very natural, gentle way to help me unearth things in my heart. A lot of times, we may not be aware of our inner thoughts and feelings. An effective mentor would help us identify them while offering guidance and encouragement. Even if they may not have all the answers, often just talking to someone relatable—someone who has been there—can make a world of difference.

A mentor is someone who sees more talent and ability within you, than you see in yourself, and helps bring it out of you.

—Bob Proctor

PAY IT FORWARD

As you become more experienced in your career or more seasoned in specific skillsets, I urge you to pay it forward and become a mentor yourself. Notice I did not say "when you get older." Mentorship is age-agnostic. True, typically, an older person mentors a younger person simply due to experience, but that is not a *rule*. I have seen phenomenal young leaders lead a great following of all ages. If you are particularly good at one subject, volunteer to become a tutor! If you have overcome a certain ordeal, lend a hand to someone going through similar brokenness. If there is an area where you can be a positive influence and pour into someone's life, be that light. You could turn someone's life around, provide more meaning and purpose, or be that springboard they need to launch into something that makes their future so much brighter. If you see someone who needs help, consider reaching out first. Recognize you were also once shy about reaching out to potential mentors and wished they had approached you first. Not everyone recognizes they need help. Remember, the worst-case scenario is they say no. How great would it be that they, in turn, go and help change more lives for the better?

BE BOLD WITH YOUR ASK
PAUL'S STORY

Years ago, I started out as an I.T. guy who had a passion for photography. Eventually, I realized I wanted to pursue a career as a full-time photographer, so I quit my job and went to photography school. After graduating, I found myself competing against other new graduates in Los Angeles, which was already saturated with many experienced and talented photographers. The biggest struggle for me and other new graduates was the lack of established clientele. L.A. was a scene where everyone knew someone who was a photographer, so it was particularly difficult to get started.

I was determined to make it work because I hadn't abandoned my previous job with a steady income to fail as an artist. Photographers have the power to capture precious moments in life, and I believed I could touch people's lives in this manner. However, my determination did not diminish the competitive landscape. I decided to seek opportunities to work alongside established photographers, thinking that might give me the start in the industry I needed. My mindset was if you are going to learn, go learn from the best. Plus, you never know who will say yes.

So, I boldly approached one of the top celebrity wedding photographers in L.A. at the time. Much to my surprise, he welcomed me to his team. To increase my exposure and to accelerate my path, I sought out the most renowned fashion and celebrity commercial photographer to see if he could take me in as well. I was pleasantly surprised to receive an affirmative response and learned a lot from these two famous photographers, in two very different fields within the photography industry. They opened doors that may never have been possible without their generosity. They didn't see me as competition but readily shared their platform and introduced me to influential people in the industry, not as an apprentice but as a peer.

I've had many people recognize my photography talent, that "I have an eye like no other." However, having that alone likely would not have been enough to help me build up a photography career so quickly. I needed the real-life experience, and these mentors enabled these opportunities. Sometimes, talent alone isn't enough; you need the courage to first seek out opportunities, the boldness to simply ask. Recognize people who care enough to share and don't hold yourself back from inviting them into your life. And down the road when you are in a position to pour into others, don't hesitate to do so.

Before you are a leader, success is all about growing yourself. When you become a leader, success is all about growing others.

—Jack Welch

TAKEAWAYS

- Mentors can help you with many components of your life and be that ongoing source of support and encouragement you need to keep on growing.

- Find mentors whom you respect and admire, people who inspire and challenge you.

- Pay it forward by mentoring others to help them become better versions of themselves.

14

IT'S OKAY TO FAIL

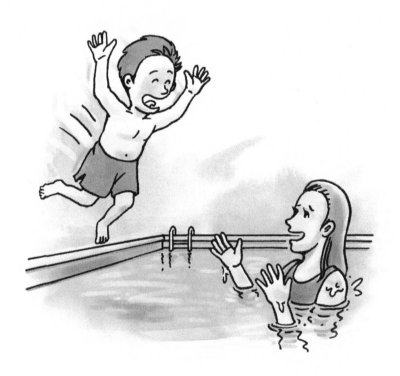

Success is not final, failure is not fatal; it is the courage to continue that counts.

—Winston Churchill

Don't hold yourself back from going for your dreams because of a fear of failing. The unknown can be scary, but it doesn't have to overwhelm you. It's okay to be scared but still give something a shot.

Failure teaches you like nothing else can. If you don't give it a try, you'll never know. It'll always be just a *what if* and *maybe I could have.*

GIVE YOURSELF THE PERMISSION TO FAIL

Failure is inevitable. If someone tells you they have never failed in their entire life, they're dishonest. Everyone fails. *Everyone.* We have all been failing since birth.

We failed plenty of times as babies. First, we learned to roll over, then to sit up, then to crawl, then to walk. Each stage took many, many tries and involved many, many tumbles. What's most admirable is not the fact that we eventually learned to walk but that we never gave up trying. We might have cried when our butts hit the ground, but I am pretty sure we got back up to try again. And then one day, we did it—we took our first step!

Sometimes, our fear of failure stems from worrying about what others think of us. As babies, we didn't care what others thought as we progressed through those developmental milestones. We just pressed on as though that's all we were meant to do—grow. We can't live life constantly overly concerned about others' approval. If these people matter in your life, chances are they would still love us regardless of how much we may fail. For everyone else, let them think whatever they want. You cannot please everyone, nor should you allow them to have that much influence over you. The more you are trying to undertake something of significance, the more haters you may encounter. If people try to make you feel small for attempting something meaningful to you, they probably aren't someone you should keep in your life anyway.

Think of all the people out there who tried and failed but kept trying. There are plenty of people in every industry in every aspect that you can consider—athletes, corporate leaders, politicians, educators, chefs, first responders, artists, entertainers, and business owners. They must have had numerous opportunities to try something but failed. But I'd bet that those who we consider successful learned from their failures and built upon them. Instead of focusing on their failures, they turned them into lessons.

It's reasonable to worry about our reputations. It's a part of us that makes us feel esteemed and valued. Most of us would go out of our way to protect our reputations. And perhaps that's why as babies, we pressed on with our mobility development because we weren't preoccupied with trying not to look foolish. There was no shame, no embarrassment. We wanted to get better and master one more skill. Of course, perhaps having cheerleaders—regardless of how ridiculous

IT'S OKAY TO FAIL

we looked waddling around like drunks as we took our first steps—helped encourage us to keep trying.

You may catch yourself holding back from trying something you consider worthwhile. Maybe you think: *If only it didn't threaten my reputation.* Now, think of the last person you know whose reputation was ruined permanently because of something they did or tried. Is this someone you know or a world-renowned figure? How many people do you think remember the incident and all of its details? There isn't a whole lot one can do that will cause irreparable damage to one's name. Weigh that against what you are trying to accomplish. Now, consider whether this fear is really what your mind is setting it out to be.

We can overcome fear. Don't ignore it, but don't feed it either. Don't give it more power. If what you want to do is good—good for you, good for others—then tell yourself this: *Sure, I'm scared, but I can do it anyway.*

> *There is no courage without fear.*
>
> —Hua Zhou from *Mulan*

When we are mindful that failure is a necessary step to accomplish our goals, we stop giving it the spotlight. We stop exaggerating its importance, its authority. Think of failure as nothing more than being part of the process. It's simply trial and error.

And we have had quite a bit of practice already. We know how to fail, but we also have experience in getting back up and trying again.

GET PERSPECTIVE

No one expects you to do everything perfectly every time. So, don't set that as an expectation for yourself. Even professional athletes don't get perfect scores every time they play. Part of the fun is in the learning process and in getting better at what we do.

Keep in mind that others may be equally—if not more—afraid to fail. You likely are not the only one who doesn't feel 100% confident all the time. The difference is in what you do with the fear.

I have sat in on presentations where a speaker appeared nervous, their voice shaky. It always surprises me when I witness this. To me, I am *always* the one who is the least prepared, the least qualified, the one with the greatest stage fright. I am always *so sure* everyone can detect my nerves (like sharks smelling blood!) and hear the tremble in my voice. And at least a couple of times, I lost my train of thought and rambled, and my face got all flushed from the embarrassment. Yet time and again, I received compliments about my presentations.

Truthfully, I am still learning to become a better speaker, something I'm sure I will continue to work on beyond my retirement. My point is, we are often our biggest critic, and while it may help us sustain a desire to improve, it can handicap us by diminishing our self-confidence. When getting ready to speak in front of an audience, there is a big difference between thinking: *I will deliver a message that will help them,* and thinking: *I will make a fool out of myself, and everyone is going to think this is the biggest waste of their time.* If you go in with a failing mindset, you're not setting yourself up for success.

Even if you make a mistake, know that it's okay. So what if I tripped on my words and ended up giving a less-than-perfect

159

presentation? Yes, it's not ideal, but it's not the end of the world either. Instead of throwing my hands up and declaring *I'm done*, it encouraged me to prepare even better next time. I rehearsed double the amount compared to the previous time and observed myself speaking in the mirror. Perhaps next time I should practice in front of a friend or even record a video of my presentation to improve my body language. The thought of watching a video of myself speaking makes me cringe, but it should be no different than a golfer watching videos of his swings, all for improvement, one slight adjustment at a time.

Remember this: don't let failure define you. Even if you failed at something, no matter how severe it may be, it's only *your attempt* that may have not succeeded. It doesn't make *you* a failure.

The only thing worse than starting something and failing is not starting something.

—Seth Godin

HAVE A PLAN AND BE PREPARED

We may be less apprehensive about the possibility of failure if we anticipate it. That's not a suggestion to *plan* to fail. No, don't *plan* to fail! But know that sometimes for us to succeed, there will be trials and tribulations. We need to face them head-on, create a plan to tackle them, and keep advancing. So, when we prepare for the chance that things may not go as smoothly as we want them to, we wouldn't be surprised and can recompose ourselves faster.

Sometimes the fear of uncertainty, rather than the fear of failure, is what cripples us. The *what-ifs* make us afraid to make a move. In those cases, consider the worst-case scenario—what is the worst that can happen? Visualize it to make it more real. If it's not that bad, then really, you do not need to be afraid of your worst fear. It might be unsettling to press on, but at least you know that even if the absolute worst were to happen, it's nothing you cannot bear.

GET SUPPORT

Having support from people who can cheer you on can make a huge difference. If you are interested in trying but are afraid of taking that first step, find someone to encourage you and hold you accountable. It can be someone who has experience in that specific area or someone who could be your sidekick. Let's say you want to start a new business venture and ultimately be an entrepreneur and your own boss. But perhaps the thought of departing from a corporate job with a steady income seems too risky. At the same time, you feel a pull to do something on your own.

Support can appear in different forms to help steer you closer to your goal while alleviating your anxiety and fears.

1. Engage in literature and webinars that focus on helping people start businesses. There is a ton of information out there to leverage. For inspiration, you may be able to get your hands on case studies to understand what obstacles others on a similar journey faced and what their solutions were.

2. Find a friend who you consider to be a successful entrepreneur. If you don't personally know someone like that, ask around for referrals. Someone must know someone within two or three degrees of separation. Pick their brain, ask for guidance, and seek their advice for your business idea. Use them as a sounding board. You will learn so much in the process. They may be able to identify pitfalls and opportunities that you may miss otherwise. Leverage their experience and skills to help you stay focused on your ultimate goal and not get sidetracked by fears and worries.

3. Hire a business coach or consultant. This may be an expensive option, but sometimes customized one-on-one help is what we need. It could also be a more efficient way to get you to where you want to be, especially if you have a relatively short timeline.

A WINNER'S COURAGE
ALAN'S STORY

Shortly after starting my freshman year of high school, the Student Council announced the upcoming elections for two freshman representative positions. Even though school had only recently started, there was already some popularity competition. Soon, there were banners up from candidates running for Student Council. One unexpected candidate appeared—a petite, humble, quiet guy you wouldn't envision running for a leadership position. His banner had the cheesiest slogan of all. It was so tacky that it became an everyday joke. People greeted him in the hallway with his slogan. People muttered it under their breaths to trigger a snicker or two. But guess what? It stood out, and people remembered it. And the most admirable part was he played along with it. I recall wondering how he could be so thick-skinned not to let all the mockery bother him. But perhaps that comes with the territory. You want your peers to select you as class rep; you need to be prepared not everyone will vote for you.

All the candidates made their final speeches in a forum with over 500 ninth graders. I don't recall much of the exact words, but I remember how impressed I was by this guy's message. It wasn't particularly captivating, but it was apparent that he knew it was a long shot to go for Student Council; his chance was slimmer than all the other candidates. He recognized he didn't have the presence or stature of a leader that he believed most of the class looked for, but he gave his word to us that he would represent us to the best of his abilities if elected. He highlighted his courage to take on whatever challenges this position might entail. Knowing how he wasn't a favorite candidate, merely being there showed incredible bravery.

He didn't win the election.

However, I think he gained a lot from that experience. He found a way to push aside his fear, went after his dream, allowed himself to be a laughingstock for *months* over a silly slogan, and he never publicly appeared to be troubled by it. That is a distinct indication of strength. He showed that sometimes, it's by laughing *with others at yourself* that you not let people get to you nor taint your reputation. He demonstrated that despite not fitting the preconception of a model leader, he would work harder to persuade people he had what it took to do the job. As a small little guy holding a microphone in the middle of a big space with over 500 expressionless faces staring at him, he showed courage and didn't let fear consume him. He gained a lot of respect and new, genuine friendships after that season. People saw him for who he was—a nice, humble, authentic guy you would want as a friend. They finally stopped mocking his slogan.

He may not have won the position, but he certainly won in the person he became, the character he built.

Consider the fire that was in him, that carried him through that whole process. Passion propelled him as he focused on his goal, and he didn't get distracted by the setbacks, the ridiculing. He didn't let others' public opinions discourage him. And he certainly did not allow fear to stop him from trying in the first place.

As a ninth grader, that fire could carry him far along in life. If he could figure out that early on, as a fourteen-year-old, to overcome his fears and not let them hold him back, there is really no limit to what he could do.

I learned that courage was not the absence of fear, but the triumph over it. The brave man is not he who does not feel afraid, but he who conquers that fear.

—Nelson Mandela

TAKEAWAYS

- Give yourself permission to fail.

- Understand your fear and what's holding you back. Seek support and encouragement to be part of your journey.

- Plan for the worst-case scenario so you are prepared and to loosen the grip fear has on you.

15

LEARN TO LOVE TO LEARN

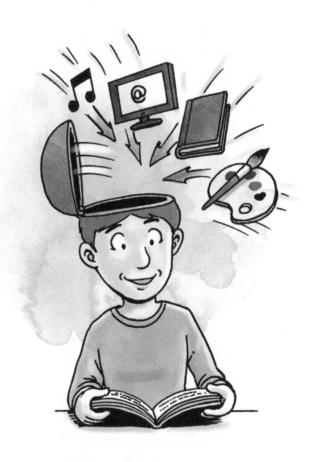

The capacity to learn is a gift; the ability to learn is a skill; the willingness to learn is a choice.

—Brian Herbert

James was a help desk agent for an Internet service provider. One day, he picked up a call from a customer who asked to cancel his Internet service. When James asked the customer why, the customer matter-of-factly stated, "because I have read everything on the Internet." This claim dumbfounded James, but the customer was serious. He truly believed he had consumed everything the Internet had to offer. After some more questioning, James realized the customer had finished reading one particular website and the associated links. James proceeded to introduce Google, and after doing some sample searches, the customer realized he had more to read on the Internet and no longer wanted to disconnect his service.

When I first heard this story, I had a good laugh. Extreme as this was, we are taking a similar stance if we close our minds to learning new things. There is so much to learn in life. You may be surprised by the exposure you haven't yet had and how much is out there to pique your interest. It merely requires an open mind.

If we don't keep learning, we become stagnant. Make learning a lifetime goal. It will keep your mind fresh, your attitude receptive, your outlook curious. Learning doesn't end with school. Those who adapt well to change want to learn as change goes on—and let's face it, change is inevitable.

Change happens every day! Everything moves forward and progresses—your friends, technology, the world. Choosing to stay put in your current frame of mind means choosing not to grow along with everyone else. It may not be long before you find yourself relatively obsolete. If you work with the younger generation as a parent, coach, or teacher, it's even more necessary to keep learning, to keep up with the young ones so that you can understand things from their lens.

Some people love formal education, and some cannot wait for the end of school so they can be *free*. Suppose you relate more with the latter group. In that case, I encourage you to separate the concept of learning from a formal school setting with a predetermined curriculum, to an enjoyable experience when you decide what you want to learn on your terms. Learning a new skill or a new hobby is very different than sitting in a classroom trying to absorb all the knowledge presented to you. So, if school didn't excite you, don't write off learning in general. Push to continue to grow and expand your horizon in one way or another. *Learn* to love to learn.

Sometimes, we may recognize there is still much to learn but believe we are too busy. That, too, is a similar argument. This is not to downplay anyone's busyness, but the fact is, everyone is busy. It's just how we prioritize the use of our time.

LEARN TO FOSTER A NEW LOVE

If you don't already enjoy the process of learning new things, then the first step is to figure out how to become excited to learn something new.

To start nurturing this interest, start with something simple or something you are already slightly curious about. Then, intentionally set out to explore. It's hard to truly *know* whether something is enjoyable without actually trying it out. You can start by making a list of your likes and dislikes. You may find you are great at something you didn't realize.

When I was in my early twenties, I was among a circle of friends who all knew how to make a few signature dishes. I felt inept in comparison like I was the only one who brought the takeout dishes, ready-to-eat dessert, or, the easiest of all, beverages. But the more lacking I felt, the more I pushed myself to explore easy recipes. It didn't quite stem from the desire to say I could also cook, but more because my friends made cooking seem so fun that I felt like I was missing out. I tried making salad dressings, simple appetizers, and easy desserts, and soon I felt that I could attend these potluck gatherings as an equal. None of my friends ever cared that I wasn't bringing homemade stuff. They certainly didn't love me less. But it was from observing and learning from them that I could uncover a knack for putting together a few signature dishes myself. Sure, the first few tries weren't exactly stellar, but they appreciated my efforts all the same. It was through their positive attitude that I felt encouraged to keep trying. That one bad batch didn't mean that's all I could cook. I could have given up early on after the first dish was too salty, too sweet, or outright burnt. But those obvious areas were usually the easiest to fix. After all, acknowledgment is the first step. So, if it's too salty, put in less salt. Too sweet? Put in less sugar. Too burnt? Well, cook it less next time.

LEARN TO NOT HOLD BACK (FOR THE WRONG REASONS)

If childhood trauma, self-esteem, timidity, or a shyer personality keeps you from trying new things, you can do it without alerting others. You're not obligated to tell anyone.

Keep in mind everyone learns at different paces and styles. What may seem natural to someone may not be as natural to someone else. Don't take that as a sign that you can *never* do well. It just means you have some work to do before you get there. Remember, failures don't define you. Use them as stepping stones and build upon them.

Sometimes, learning can feel unpleasant and exhausting. However, it shouldn't. One way around it is to find good teachers who are passionate about what you are trying to learn and teach in an engaging and effective manner. Some people are so natural at teaching and can make the most boring topic fascinating. I had a chemistry teacher in high school who could break down different components so well; the concepts were easy to grasp and easy to apply. Conversely, I had a physics teacher who read out the textbook with no further explanation. Perhaps you can guess which subject I enjoyed more and scored higher on.

Another way is to find a learning partner. Having a buddy can make it more fun. I know friends who take cooking classes together and have a blast each time. Others have friends who hold each other accountable to learn something new. It can be very interesting to hear what others have learned. That might also give you ideas on what to explore next!

Make learning a habit, an insatiable craving. *Learn to love to learn* early on. Let learning become a part of you, a part of your ongoing curiosity. It will help you to think differently, more creatively, and innovatively. You will get better at challenging yourself to learn something new and do something different. You will become more comfortable with being uncomfortable. And that becomes a skill, a level of confidence to help you for the rest of your life.

Seek to learn constantly while you live; do not wait in the faith that old age by itself will bring wisdom.

—Solon

EXPAND YOUR HORIZONS

Need some ideas to get started?

- Try a new food place. If you are unsure what to order, the servers can provide some recommendations. If you're not quite ready for that, then the next time you're at your most frequented restaurant, try a new dish. Switch things up.

- If you have a typical route to school or work, pick a different route on a random day. If there is only one path to getting there, then when you have an extra fifteen minutes, spend it to take a detour. I've lived in the same neighborhood for several years now and still am not familiar with all the small streets in my area.

- Pick up a new instrument.

- Take vocal lessons. (So many of you should be singing for people and not just in the shower!)

- Learn to draw. Many people lose *touch with* their creativity as they get older; they don't lose their creativity altogether. When we were little kids, we came up with all sorts of creative art. Somehow as we aged, we became more critical of ourselves and felt we should maintain some standard or else stop. Well, wake up that creative side and start drawing. It'd open up a whole new world. Take some drawing classes, look up online art tutorials, or find an artist friend who can teach you some techniques to get started. Giving the right brain some prime time can give you new perspectives on things you normally do with your left brain.

- Get to know acquaintances better. We say hello to so many people, but we can learn something new about them—what do they like to do for fun? What is their favorite food? Were they born and raised locally, or did they move here from somewhere else? You may realize you share more things in common than you think. Or you may discover their interests, and that's also good.

- Travel. If traveling makes you feel apprehensive, start somewhere close for three to four days. As you venture out, see new things, experience new culture, and try new food, you will likely want to venture further. One thing that helps is an adventurous travel companion. If you are starting, go with someone or a group who knows what they are doing. Don't entirely rely on them to do all the research; there is much to learn from the research process alone. Or, as a start, join a tour that will alleviate some of the anxiety of unfamiliar traveling.

- Meet new people—people can teach us so much. We tend to gravitate toward those who are similar to us, but it's fun to meet individuals we wouldn't normally hang with. Take the time to learn about them because everyone has a story. What's theirs?

- Move out of your city, state, province, or even your country. If you're a student, find an exchange program that could give you this opportunity. If you're currently working and employed by a big company, explore ways to work at a different location. If that option is not available, research companies you may want to work for and apply. It might be a long shot, but your skillset and courage might be what they are looking for.

- Go volunteer. Get involved with non-profit organizations; they can always use more help.

- Use your skills to teach someone something. You may be surprised by how your perspective changes when you assume the role of a teacher. It may further expand *your* knowledge in this area to continue teaching your student something new and exciting. So, you could very well be learning something at the same time you're teaching. This has happened to me before. During that time, I learned faster and with more depth than I recall ever learning.

If you want to be a parent in the future, gain exposure to kids early on. Find ways to be more familiar with raising children, even if it's babysitting or volunteering at church; working alongside kids will help you understand them so much better. It's rather ironic, but kids can teach you so much. But first, we need to keep our eyes, hearts, and minds open and be ready to learn.

BLESSING OTHERS
MY STORY

Growing up, I had always relied on my mom to help me sew, replace buttons, hem my pants, anything that involved a needle and thread. One day, she shared with me she was glad she took the time to learn to sew when she was young. Allow me to point out that when my mom was young, there was no Internet, no YouTube tutorials, and no Facebook videos to look up. She had to look for in-person options that were well within her budget and still allowed her to learn comprehensively. She had to improvise a lot because she wasn't paying for an entire course; her financial situation at the time didn't allow for formal classes. This semi-self-taught skill turned out to serve her and her family as she grew up and her future husband and children. Not only that, but through her sewing and knitting, she was able to be a blessing to others. Therefore, regarding what she would tell her younger self, she felt proud she had pushed herself to become proficient at sewing. The biggest fruit this bore was that she was able to make things with love and her own hands for her family to wear.

Later on in life, friends and relatives expressed appreciation for something my mom made for them years ago—tote bags, handknitted sweaters, winter hats, scarves—things she had long forgotten. Though it wasn't something she necessarily remembered, the fact that other people were still thanking her so many years later showed how much these gifts meant to them. They recognized the hands and love behind the items. Her persistence to learn how to sew paid off in the many hearts she touched.

Anyone who stops learning is old, whether this happens at twenty or eighty. Anyone who keeps on learning not only remains young but becomes constantly more valuable—regardless of physical capacity.

—Henry Ford

TAKEAWAYS

- Foster a love for learning and stay curious. It'll keep things interesting for the rest of your life.

- Don't hold back from learning for the wrong reasons.

- Explore something new on a regular basis. Meet new people, try new food, or visit a new place.

16

BE KIND, UNCONDITIONALLY

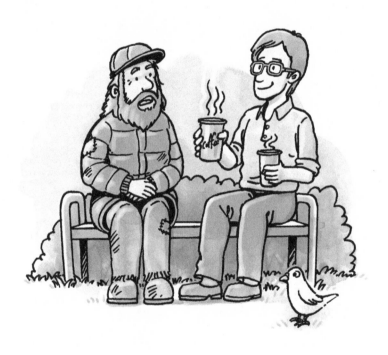

Kind words can be short and easy to speak, but their echoes are truly endless.

—Mother Teresa

We live in a harsh world. Every day we hear bad news of some type from somewhere—cruelty, racism, war, conflict, hatred, and anger. Unfortunately, some value themselves above others rather than a greater good and aren't willing to put others' well-being first. But let's face it, we all tend to be selfish to some extent. It's practically impossible to *always* put others first.

There is kindness in the world; I am sure of it. But there isn't enough. If more of us displayed acts of love and kindness more often, no matter how small, the ripple effect could change the world. Our choosing to be kind can cover the earth with compassion and love.

BE KIND TO OTHERS

Being kind is one of those things that's easy to say but hard to do, especially if we were to do it consistently. And why? Is it because it's not within our nature to be good?

Do we typically act first from a heart of kindness or a heart of selfishness? When we do something kind for others, is it an automatic response or something we convince ourselves that we *have* to do?

How can we shape our heart so that it genuinely wants to be kind and takes the initiative?

Oftentimes, we assume the worst in people. When we hear *something happened* or *somebody did such-and-such,* we tend to assume ill intentions when we don't know all the details.

Give others the benefit of the doubt. If you need to assume anything, try to assume the best about people. There is hardly anyone who isn't struggling with something in their life at any given time. Their smiles could very well be a disguise. If you think you understand everything going on in their lives and all that they are going through, chances are you're wrong. And even if they *seem* to be living the perfect life, it doesn't mean they are less deserving of kindness.

SERVE OTHERS

Be generous because you can. Give what you can, regardless of how much you feel the other person deserves. Use your talents, gifts, and resources to make a difference in someone's life. The $20 you spend on coffee each week can help feed a family for a day or two. You don't have to deprive yourself of all your indulgences, but occasionally sacrificing some of your treats to assist others can bring an unparalleled sense of joy.

Serve others without needing anything in return, even if it's just recognition. Help others anonymously. It puts an extra spark in your heart.

I once heard a story about a man taking a stroll with his son when they came across a homeless man sitting on the sidewalk.

181

There was a small, battered box in front of the man with a few coins in it. Other passersby probably dropped those in earlier that day, but it was definitely not enough to buy anything to eat. The father stopped to pull out a $100 bill from his wallet and gently placed it in the box. The man stared at it in disbelief; his eyes misted up as he lifted his face toward his donor. The father gave a tender smile with a subtle nod of his head and proceeded with his walk.

The son quickly asked his dad, "How do you know he really needs the money? How do you know he won't use it for alcohol or drugs? $100 is a lot of money to give away like that!"

"Son, what he does with the money is up to him. He can choose to do good with it or not. That's on him. But if I have the means to help him and I choose to walk by, then that says a lot more about my character."

Great opportunities to help others seldom come, but small ones surround us every day.

—Sally Koch

FORGIVE

Be generous not only with your time and money but also with your grace. Forgive quickly and forgive often. Everyone makes mistakes. Whether honest or intentional, we may hurt someone in the process and rob others of their trust in us. It may make them question their love for us.

We are no different. When we make a mistake and cause someone pain, we, too, would want to be forgiven.

Forgiveness isn't free. It might not have an attached price tag, but it does require less of an ego, less anger, and three simple yet substantial words: "I forgive you." These words require selflessness to not focus on the ache of *our* broken heart but to open it up and graciously tell the other person: "Despite what happened, despite the sorrow it caused, I choose to pardon you of this wrongdoing."

Forgiveness is liberating for both parties. It is a sense of relief for the forgiver, like a loosening knot, releasing anger and renewing the heart. For the forgiven, an unshackled feeling of a paid debt.

My best friend taught me one of the most impactful nuggets of wisdom: It's good to quickly forgive, for everyone involved. If their mistake was an honest mistake, they deserve a second chance. If they intentionally hurt you, it is not worth letting the anger eat you up and callous your heart. My friend explained holding a grudge typically bothers you more than it bothers the other person. Chances are, they may soon forget about the incident. Or worse, they may be oblivious you felt faulted against to begin with. You could very well end up more bitter than the other person.

This wisdom came from my best friend when she was eight years old! It surfaced when I asked her how she never appeared to be upset with people.

"Why bother? It's not worth it."

Holding a grudge doesn't make you strong; it makes you bitter. Forgiving doesn't make you weak; it sets you free.

—Dave Willis

BE KIND TO YOURSELF

Of all the people you will live with in your life, the longest one you will have spent time with is *yourself*. So, learn to love yourself. Don't be your harshest critic.

Don't beat yourself up over mishaps. To err is human. To not learn from them is the bigger mistake. There is a significant difference between being a narcissist versus knowing how to take good care of yourself. Don't be arrogant. Rather, be gracious.

Listen to the way you talk to yourself. Is it loving? Is it uplifting? Do you speak like an ally or an adversary? Would a good friend speak that way to you? When you look in the mirror, do you see an endless catalog of blemishes and imperfections? Or are you able to see past that and recognize the strength and beauty within? Our brightness shines from the inside. Don't conceal it with layers of makeup and merciless critique.

Your worth isn't in how many heads you turn. If you are kind and confident, beauty comes naturally. Your light will attract, not merely your appearance. People would want to be around you because of who you are.

Take good care of yourself psychologically and spiritually. Don't bottle up your emotions, expecting them to work themselves out. Expose them, talk about them, address them. Learn to overcome, not just *get over* but *go through* the painful circumstances. Find support through family, friends, or professional resources. Pride is not important enough to deny yourself the benefits of help. Come out a better, stronger version of you. You may find your experiences can help others face similar ordeals in the future.

BE GRATEFUL

Say thank you often and sincerely. Don't assume people know. It could be the smallest deed, but taking a second to show our appreciation can go a long way.

Whether something deserves a thank you depends on our perspective. Not everyone expects thanks for everything they do, but it sure would be nice, wouldn't it? How many times do you think a janitor receives thanks? Probably not often. Yet they work consistently day in and day out. Their service *each* day deserves a thank you. We all expect the bathrooms clean every day, don't we? Just because you thanked them one time doesn't mean you shouldn't extend another thank you.

Likewise, take a moment to thank those who serve you regularly. Parents who cook your meals, your spouse who continues to put your needs first, friends who stand by you, children who tolerate your moods, workers who collect your trash, civil workers who keep the city running, school staff who ensure your children are educated and safe. Appreciate them like rainbows. Every time a rainbow illuminates the sky, we still admire it with a new sense of awe, as though it is the first rainbow we have ever seen. Growing up in Hawai'i, where rainbows appear practically every day during winter because of the frequent rainfalls, my children have seen countless rainbows. Yet, they still gasp at the sight of each one with authentic wonder. And my husband and I still fumble for our phones, hoping to catch a snapshot of it before it disappears, even though we may already have captured dozens of photos of rainbows. Each rainbow on its own is special. Similarly, no matter how many times someone does something for you, even if it's part of their role or job, show continuous appreciation.

THE UNKNOWNS BENEATH THE SURFACE
SUSIE'S STORY

It was Thursday of a grueling, exhausting work week. Everyone had worked more than twelve hours each day for the previous two weeks. While in a meeting, I asked for clarification about something on a project, and Anna explained. But a few minutes later, I was still confused and asked again. Anna's angry response made me realize I had probably repeated my question more times than that and wore out her patience.

"I already answered that question. Can you pay attention so you aren't wasting everyone's time?"

I apologized and kept quiet the rest of the meeting. My brain was foggy from extreme sleep deprivation. I tried to stay focused on the project, but my mind kept wandering to my daughter, hoping she was feeling better, recovering in the hospital from her injury the other night. I hadn't shared it with the team; everyone had enough to worry about after all, racing against the clock to launch the project on time.

Even after Anna's outburst, I chose not to tell the team about my daughter. I didn't want to come across as making excuses or for them to feel obligated to take on my work.

A couple of weeks went by and somehow, the team caught word of my daughter's condition. Anna felt awful for how she treated me. She wished I had shared my circumstances with the team so they could be more understanding of what I was going through. It was as though she knew she would have reacted differently to my repetitive questions had she been aware of my struggles.

But why did it require a hospitalized daughter to nudge someone to be kind? Shouldn't we treat people with grace and respect because it's the right thing to do and not because we pity them for their unfortunate circumstances?

After that incident, I became much more conscious about the assumptions I made about people and tried my best to always give others the benefit of the doubt.

The best thing to give to your enemy is forgiveness; to an opponent, tolerance; to a friend, your heart; to your child, a good example; to a father, deference; to your mother, conduct that will make her proud of you; to yourself, respect; to all men, charity.

—Arthur James Balfour

TAKEAWAYS

- Be kind to others and develop a serving heart.
- Be kind to yourself; there are enough critics in the world.
- Be forgiving and be grateful.

17

FIRST, BE THE RIGHT ONE

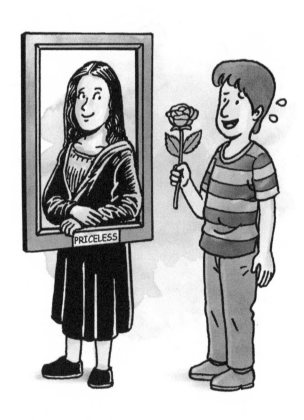

Become the person the person you're looking for is looking for.

—Andy Stanley

Most of us invest so much time thinking and agonizing over *finding the right one* that we often overlook the importance of first working on ourselves so that we can *be* the right one for our "Mr. Right" or "Mrs. Right."

We need to first be the right one.

We cannot control another's character, traits, or behaviors, but we can do something about ours and what we ultimately bring to our marriage.

Just as you may have specific criteria for your spouse, others have criteria for theirs too. And before we commit ourselves as someone's lifelong partner, there are certain things we can do to make sure we are putting our best foot forward and not only counting on *receiving* from the other party.

I'm not talking about things that make you who you are, such as your values, personality, and appearance. Rather, I'm talking about the things we can improve.

Don't get me wrong; no one is perfect. This is not a suggestion to aim for perfection. But if we're truthful with ourselves, there are attributes we can further develop and further refine. Are we self-centered? Are we judgmental? Do we manage our anger well? Are we patient? Are we kind?

One of the best guiding posts I can think of for an optimal character comes from the book of Galatians in the Bible—the fruits of the Spirit:

- Love

- Joy

- Peace

- Patience

- Kindness

- Goodness

- Faithfulness

- Gentleness

- Self-Control[2]

It may be bold of me to suggest one more quality: humility.

Give yourself an honest evaluation of where you are with these traits. Better yet, ask a few close friends or family members and let them evaluate you. How others perceive us from the outside could drastically differ from how we view ourselves. We may think we're loving, but if people around us don't seem to agree with that, then that should make a statement. Permit them to be authentic, to be real with you. After all, that's what you need (even if it may not be what you want), right?

Think of those in your social circle. Picture someone close to living those nine virtues. What are they like? What sets them apart?

I can easily picture a few of my friends with sincere, self-less, authentic, genuinely wanting-the-best-for-you kind of

---

[2] New Living Translation Bible. 2015. Galatians 5:22-23.

love. They are equally patient with their parents as they are with their kids. Their kindness reaches out to strangers and friends alike. They don't weigh what they give against what they may receive in return; they shield their financial status by their humility, uphold their riches by their generosity, and show compassion toward others.

And yet they are the same people who don't consider themselves too good for improvement. They see themselves as imperfect, as needing growth and grace.

Again, the purpose isn't to perfect ourselves before we are engaged or married. If that was the case, we'd have a whole world of single people. (And if anyone tries to argue that their partner is absolutely perfect, you may not have been together long enough!) It is most important to recognize we are all works-in-progress; there is much to cultivate. Your future spouse is worthwhile and needs you to keep striving to be better, whether you have met them yet or not.

GATHER WISDOM BEFORE YOU NEED IT

A friend of mine, now well in his forties, once mentioned he invested one year to read as many books about marriage as possible.

He was twenty.

And single.

I can think of so much more for a twenty-year-old single guy to be doing than sitting at home reading marriage books. However, he knew he wanted to get married one day and wanted it to be a healthy and successful marriage. He also knew he wanted children and believed they'd deserve a loving home. He recognized he didn't know much about what made marriages last but knew how common divorces were and didn't want that to happen to him in the future. So, he set out to best equip himself to become a spouse worth marrying. He armed himself with as much knowledge as possible about building a strong marriage and understanding challenges and pitfalls.

He understood how critical it was to get ahead by first learning what he needed *before* he went on his pursuit for that special someone.

To say I was impressed would be an understatement. He showed wisdom beyond his years. It's so important to prepare ourselves with the proper knowledge *before* we need it. Just like school educates us before joining the workforce and a doctor receives extensive training before performing medical duties, (can you imagine a surgeon trying to conduct a real-life surgery while following an open textbook!) my friend's approach made so much sense, but it's uncommon. Couples typically engage in premarital counseling after their engagement, if at all. The few months of *training* represents just a little sliver of time compared to the number of years— *decades*—the marriage is *meant* to last.

LET THE PAST BE THE PAST

Sometimes, we carry baggage from previous relationships into new ones. We should clear our hearts and minds free of all the wrongs from our exes and let those remain in our pasts. Treat each relationship as a fresh start. Dragging baggage into a new relationship can poison it before it even starts.

Find closure. The only thing to take from these past failed relationships is learning about your needs and wants, what worked and didn't, and what you cannot live with.

EXPECTATIONS

Do you have unspoken expectations of *your* spouse? What will he or she be like? What will they do for you and for the family? Do you envision an equal sharing of housework, or do you anticipate your future spouse fully taking on certain tasks around the house?

Many couples don't discuss the finer details before getting married, but it's often the little things that cause conflict and arguments. If you don't know how to cook, are you willing to learn? Do you expect your spouse to do all the cooking? Do you anticipate eating out or getting takeout every day? If you are counting on your spouse to do most of the cooking, would you be okay doing the dishes, or is the expectation that they will do that too? Would you be able to fulfill those duties with joy all the time?

Do you expect a certain lifestyle? Do you envision a dual-income household or for one of you to switch to part-time or stop working altogether when children enter the picture? Do you have expectations about time spent with your families? How will you spend the holidays?

What about parenting styles? I have seen some people expect the other spouse to do most of the disciplining. And other couples assume they will share the responsibility, yet they disagree on the approach.

People say marriages require compromises, both sides have to do their parts, and that it's a 50/50 partnership. But it's more accurate to say marriages require our all, our 100%. Marriages need spouses to think of each other as teammates playing on the same team, with a shared mission and goals. When one person is down, the other *willingly* jumps in and covers. There is no tallying of who did what or who said what. We should give grace and forgiveness generously and infinitely. Each one puts in their best to benefit the greater good—the marriage and the family. They don't give their best to other aspects of life—careers, friends, hobbies—while leaving the scraps for their spouse or children. They act out their love and treat each other with respect. They want what's best for their teammate, even if it sometimes means diminishing their own desires. They don't need to be right all the time, especially if it's at the expense of the relationship. And they don't take each other for granted.

All that is, of course, easier said than done. I would argue couples who have been married for many years still struggle some days. It's difficult to be selfless *all* the time. But we can try. We may be far from being the perfect spouse, but we can start to work toward that vision. Having the right mindset already gets you one step closer.

Are you ready to give your (future) marriage your all?

WHEN YOU DON'T LET GO
KELSEY'S STORY

My three-year-long relationship ended when I discovered my boyfriend's infidelity. I was so sure he was the one and secretly expected him to propose in the near future. My dream was shattered when I confronted him about my suspicions, and he admitted to seeing someone behind my back for a year. In hindsight, his behavior—his hot-and-cold treatments, being out of reach a lot of times but showering me with a lot of attention on special occasions as though he had to make up for something—suddenly, *it all made sense.*

Sometime later, I began a new relationship with someone else. This guy was nothing like my ex, and I was excited to welcome this new chapter of my life. A fresh start would do me a lot of good.

Soon, I realized I had a hard time trusting him. When I couldn't reach him, my imagination ran wild. No matter how hard I tried, I couldn't shake off the paranoia. I honestly shared with him about my past, justifying my lack of trust. At first, he was sympathetic about what I had gone through and understanding of my trauma. After a while, it started to take a toll on our relationship. He told me if there was no trust, there wasn't much a relationship could stand on. And the lack of trust stemmed from someone else, not because of something he did. It was as though he spent each day trying to repair a mistake someone else made. He knew it wasn't my fault, but if there was nothing he could do to fully earn my trust, he couldn't see much of a future for us to stay together.

And with that, our relationship came to an end. I was angry at him for his lack of compassion. But as I reflected further upon this last failure of a relationship, I was more frustrated with myself for my inability to start fresh, see him for who he was, and not expect him to pay the price of someone else's wrongdoings. Perhaps I wasn't ready for a new relationship until I let myself heal, so I could leave my past where it was supposed to be—behind me.

WHEN VALUES ARE MISALIGNED
GERALD'S STORY

For years, I wondered how I let my perfect one get away. She encouraged me, stood by my side, and accepted me for who I was even when my family didn't. Then, one day, she grew more distant. It probably didn't happen overnight, but I was oblivious for so long; it felt like she woke up and fell out of love with me one day.

Eventually, I learned the truth: she couldn't see the life I was trying to build included her. I had a plan meticulously laid out to continuously increase my income and join the affluent class. What I realized too late was that I had never considered what she wanted. How ironic because part of my desire to make millions was to give her a lavish lifestyle. I never asked her if that was what would make her happy. But I knew she wasn't materialistic; I was the one who was into designer names. It gave me a certain status that I craved, made me feel like I mattered. I could *finally* prove myself to all the people who looked down on me. But she just wanted a simple life, someone who would spend time with her. I was too busy to notice as I tried to make it big, working insane hours because I had convinced myself it would be through money and luxurious things that she'd understand my devotion for her. I realized I was only doing it for myself and my pride. I needed to prove my capabilities to the world.

I wasn't ready to settle down if I was honest with myself, especially not for a plain, basic life. In hindsight, my love for her wouldn't have compensated for the excitement I sought. I craved to see more of the world, to experience more new things. I only wished I had understood that about myself before wasting so much of her time *and mine.*

HAVING THE LAST WORD
TONY'S STORY

When your spouse of over thirties years becomes terminally ill and loses the slow, painful battle, many things suddenly fall into perspective. My biggest lesson was that it is *way* more important to be kind than to be right. Prolonging arguments just to have the last word and to be right is a terrible way to nurture a relationship. So often, we press on just to prove our point, to be right. It's easy to forget that we should first seek to understand and reconcile. We lash out when we feel we've been wronged, and it bruises our egos. But when we do that, we are actually driving a big wedge into our relationships.

No one likes to be wrong. But sometimes, we need to put the other person above our needs because we love them and because there is a relationship to protect. As I held my dear Emily's hand while she took her final breath, nothing else mattered, none of the arguments over the years or times when I felt like I got the last word—none of that. What mattered was she was no longer there. What mattered was I failed to seize every day to love her the way she deserved to be loved.

Everyone thinks of changing the world, but no one thinks of changing himself.

—Leo Tolstoy

TAKEAWAYS

- Find ways to make yourself a better spouse, rather than simply focusing on finding the perfect spouse.

- Let the past be the past. Don't drag baggage from old relationships into the new.

- Marriages are not 50/50 partnerships. They are a commitment that you be willing to give your 100% unconditionally.

18

KNOW WHAT YOU WANT IN A SPOUSE

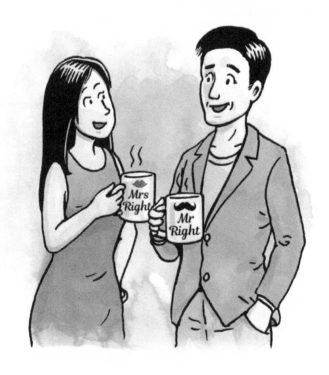

The health of your marriage tomorrow will be determined by the decisions you make today.

—Andy Stanley

Many people identify their future spouse and approach marriage by means of the sparks and passion. While affection and attraction are key ingredients for a romantic relationship, a strong marriage cannot be sustained through feelings alone. Feelings change over time and across circumstances.

When in the dating scene, girls tend to wait to be swept off their feet, and often guys may be drawn by physical appearances. If you're dating with a goal to finding your lifetime partner, it's important to see past that magnetic pull. Take the time to get a good understanding whether the person has the attributes that are important to you so you can grow a loving marriage together.

We don't just stumble into whatever job we may think is interesting and carelessly make that our career. Typically, we first assess what we enjoy doing and consider worth our time. After all, we spend much of our adult lives in our jobs. It would be tragic to not align our talents, interests, and strengths with what we do every day for a living. Without this assessment, you may end up choosing the wrong career and live with dread and regret for the rest of your life.

Similarly, with marriage, it's not wise to base it on passion alone. It's even more critical to assess what you want in your spouse, the one you will spend the rest of your life with and may become a parent of your children. Your marriage impacts practically every aspect of your life. Don't leave it to chance. It's not only about how much desire you feel for another person or how much they make your heart race. Sure, if there is no interest at all, then there may not be much to build upon, but it's not merely about the initial attraction. A lot of successful relationships started off as friendships—friends who started to realize there is romantic potential. I'm not advocating for everyone to start chasing after their friends and try turning them into romantic partners. But there is more to a love relationship than just attraction. A love relationship needs a solid foundation and two parties to join together to build something bigger and stronger. To do that, you need to first understand who would make a good partner. What qualities, when paired with yours, would make you better and them better? It's true when people say one plus one can be greater than two. It's when two people together become better than they were as individuals.

EXAMINE QUALITIES THAT MATTER TO YOU

More than likely, you have a tangible or unspoken list of qualities that you desire in your partner.

Perhaps this is a new concept to you, in which case, this is a great place to start! If you aren't sure where to begin, here is some food for thought. It's better to think about this when you're still single—when you aren't attached and clouded by feelings and emotions or have the pressure of shaping your list to fit the person you're currently dating. Re-assess as you grow older (and still unmarried) because your priorities may change. Keep in mind this list is to trigger your thought process; it is not to be an exhaustive checklist by any means.

- **Values and motivations.** If someone was primarily motivated by money, would you be okay with that? Conversely, if someone wanted to serve the community and chose to dedicate their life to non-profit, volunteer work, and were willing to compromise their quality of life, would that be okay with you? Now, these things could impact a lot of life decisions which could ultimately affect the family. Similarly, would you prefer to have an ambitious spouse who kept looking to advance their career? Or would you prefer marrying someone with a steady job, likely doing the same thing each day with little interest to advance in their career? Both have implications on how to prioritize time. The former might involve moving the family to different parts of the world, spending time away at work, missing some kids' activities, etc. But salaries could increase over the years, perhaps providing a more comfortable life for the family. The latter might be more stable; there are clearer boundaries between personal and work. The potential for pay increases might not be high, but family time might be better protected.

- **Kids.** Do you want kids? Do they want kids? Don't get into a serious relationship without sorting this one out because this is often a dealbreaker. It is nearly impossible to compromise on this—someone will need to bend, but if there are strict reasons behind their choice, it's hard to convince them otherwise. I have heard of couples who did not agree on having children but when it happened, they instantly fell in love with their newborn baby and had more children. Can you imagine if having the baby confirmed their initial decision to not want children? What kind of environment would the child grow up in? How much love would the child receive growing up? It's too much of a gamble. Have the conversation upfront.

- **Education.** This one is more for you. Don't marry someone unless you fully respect their level of education. Said another way, if any part of you could look down at someone because of their level of education, please don't get involved romantically. If they do not meet your standards, they don't deserve the burden of disappointment in your eyes.

- **Faith.** This is often another dealbreaker and not typically something compromisable, as much as you may want to believe it initially. This is foundational to a marriage because it influences your values, lifestyle, parenting approach, and how you prioritize your time. I have heard of couples with different faiths making their marriage work, and at the beginning, they agreed to let their children choose their beliefs when they got older. But until their children are at an age where they can decide, which belief would guide them? Will you, as the parent, communicate one as the *right* one without confusing them? How could they make sense out of their parents' diverging beliefs?

- **Sense of humor.** This is very important for a marriage. I have seen old couples who were still making each other laugh. There is something magical when two people share a good laugh. It helps them connect like nothing else can.

- **Key traits.** Are they kind? Are they willing to admit fault? Are they willing to change and adapt? Are they well-tempered? Are they humble? Are they agreeable? Do they listen well? How important are these things to you? Which ones are you willing to accept if you can't say yes to them all? I don't think anyone is a ten out of ten on all of these traits. It is always a give-and-take. And that's where love and acceptance come in. But what can you live with and without?

- **Spending habits.** Would you prefer a saver or a spender? It's rare to strike the perfect balance; we all tend to sway toward one or the other. A spender might feel restricted when marrying a saver. Conversely, a saver might feel frustrated over a spouse's shopping decisions. A spender marrying a spender might make saving for the family a challenge. A saver marrying a saver may yield a minimalistic life that some may view as lacking enjoyment. These are a bit extreme, but money and financial approaches are typically hot topics for many couples, so do not underestimate their power in causing conflict or keeping the peace.

- **Hobbies.** Which of your hobbies would you like to share with your partner? Which ones are you okay with not sharing?

Again, this list is a non-comprehensive list and more of a starting point to assess what's important to you in a lifelong partner. It's to help spark thoughts so you can have an honest conversation with yourself.

GET MORE CLARITY

If you have a hard time identifying what you need in a spouse, here are a few more suggestions:

- Consult with people who know you well and want the best for you. Assuming you have a good relationship with your parents and siblings, they would be a good resource for this. After all, they would want you to have a beautiful marriage, a spouse who would be a wonderful parent for their grandchildren, nieces, and nephews, and an in-law with whom they would *want* to spend time. (I have a friend who calls her mother-in-law "mother-in-love." Can you imagine how wonderful their relationship must be?) These people have known you all your life. They might even know you better than you know yourself.

- Likewise, your close friends could help. They know you and what makes you happy. Their opinions matter. Give them a platform to voice their thoughts, even if you are already dating someone. Deep down, you will know if their opinions are valid.

- Envision your life in five, ten, twenty years. How do you want your life and marriage? What kind of spouse can you imagine yourself *happily* coming home to? Would you still be excited to spend time with them?

- If you want children in the future, what kind of father or mother would you want for them? Who would be a good role model for your children to look up to?

It's important to emphasize here that I am not suggesting you ignore the element of love when selecting your spouse. Rather, I urge you not to *only* consider the element of love. Of course, we need to love the other person deeply to have them in our lives for years to come. Though some cultures might not permit one to choose their spouse, we *do* have that freedom for the most part.

Sometimes, people jump in with both feet despite intuitively knowing it's not the right thing to do. I have heard of people getting divorced in as little as a month after their wedding. Something made them want to go through with their wedding vows, perhaps in trying to avoid the embarrassment of calling a wedding off, but deep down, they knew getting married would be a huge mistake.

Love is a tricky thing. It can make us fall for the wrong person. We can see absolutely no future with the other person yet continue to stay with them because we love and care about them. But if we *really* listen to our heart and give our mind some airtime to speak up, we know it's a dead end. Sometimes couples break up, realizing there is no hope for their relationship before the wedding. Other times, it's after they get married. Sometimes, it's after children enter the picture.

Several people wished they could tell their younger selves to be braver, dare to walk away sooner when with the wrong person, listen to friends and family, and listen to themselves.

When it comes to finding the perfect spouse, remember this: *Do not settle.* This is one of the most common pieces of marriage advice. Considering marriage is meant to last a lifetime, it makes sense to practice sound judgment when selecting our life partner. Use sound judgment with a clear head.

Sometimes, things emerge as you spend more time with someone. And yes, people can change. But don't invest so much of your life and emotions as a gamble on someone's ability and willingness to change. If you don't see the qualities and values you consider as must-haves in a lifelong partner, don't prolong the pain. Don't marry someone based on what you see as their potential or your vision of who they might be. Both you and the other person deserve better. You shouldn't be with someone while constantly waiting for a better version of them to *eventually* show up. And they shouldn't be with someone who can't truly love, appreciate, and accept them as they are. If you want to believe that they will change, then let them change first. Let them show you what they can become before further commitment. You may find out that it's not what you had imagined.

WHEN MR. RIGHT MAY NOT BE THE RIGHT ONE
EMMA'S STORY

I was one of those who knew John was Mr. Right after several dates. He made me feel . . . *special*. Of all the guys I had dated in the past, none showed his admiration quite so genuinely. We had butterflies in our stomachs when we were together (or at least I wanted to believe that he did too). Often, we hopped on the phone as soon as he dropped me off at home after dinner, and we tirelessly chatted until the sun came up. Bliss was our caffeine.

We got engaged and married within a year of our first hello because we were *in love*.

It wasn't long before our marriage turned rocky. We thought things would get better after having a baby, but it just made things worse. Sure, we were completely in love with our child, but it soon became apparent that the only time we shared a smile or a laugh was when we talked about our baby. It seemed like we, as a couple, had drifted apart.

I confided in a couple of close friends who both had solid, flourishing marriages, and they assured me this was normal. According to them, marriages tend to take a backseat when children enter the picture, making the couple feel distant from each other. Shortly after, John and I had our second child. I thought this would help the family be more cohesive, but the disconnection only worsened. He felt so out of reach that I couldn't even bring up my concern of how far apart we seemed. We were tending to the kids and never to each other. There was no more passion, no more romance. I felt my marriage slipping away and didn't know what to do about it. My friends told me things would get better when the kids got older and became more independent because somehow, we would find time for each other again.

I thought I would ask: *Won't it be too late by then?* But for whatever reason, I couldn't get that question past the lump in my throat.

Even though I never asked my friends that question, I eventually learned the answer. John and I got divorced when our older child turned six. Did I ever expect to get divorced? No. I had heard people jokingly say, "After spending so much on a wedding, why would anyone get divorced?" Our wedding spared no expense. Every detail was extravagant. I got my fairy tale wedding, but it was not a happily ever after.

After going through a rather long grieving process full of anger, disappointment, denial, and guilt, I reached back out to my two good friends. They had patiently waited for my reappearance from my self-imposed dark cave. I was ashamed in so many ways that I didn't quite know how to carry myself in social situations, so I had chosen to go into isolation. Plus, wallowing in grief didn't make me the most fun person to be around.

My friends tried to keep things *normal*, but it wasn't possible. My new normal was a broken home, juggling the kids' schedules between two homes, trying to find a balance between properly disciplining the kids and spoiling them because I had limited time with them.

During a very casual conversation over coffee, Sally suddenly asked, "What was it about John that made you want to marry him?"

She hadn't intended to, but her question certainly hit a nerve.

Suddenly, everything made sense. As I fumbled for words, I realized I didn't know much about John when we got engaged and then married after four months. It just felt right, and he treated me well. *He made me feel special. We were in love.*

In hindsight, I realized feeling special is hardly a reason to marry someone. We built our marriage upon feelings, as real as they seemed. And the love we felt wasn't long-lasting enough to see us through our seventh wedding anniversary.

We had exceptionally little common ground. Sure, people say opposites attract, but how long can opposite traits and interests sustain a relationship? At first, it might seem intriguing, but opposites and differences can soon feel more like conflict. Maybe it's more reflective of time spent apart, each doing their own thing. If one person loves to hike and the other person does not even enjoy the outdoors, you can guess how many times they would hike together before they decide to spend their time separately. While it's true that couples should maintain their interests and individual time with friends, they also need interests they can enjoy together to build their relationship.

Sally shared that she knew what she needed and wanted in a husband before she seriously dated anyone. She literally had a list. My younger self would have laughed at the concept of a list.

What are we, shopping for a car? I could almost hear my younger self say.

But this grown-up, recovered-divorcee-me could now appreciate the importance of such a list. It can be a physical list on paper or a simple mental understanding of what you want in a significant other. If there are key features, must-haves, and nice-to-haves for a car that you'd likely keep for five to ten years, why wouldn't you give even more thought to your list of desired features for a spouse who is supposed to share the rest of your life with you? Yes, it's important to have that real and authentic love; your relationship needs that. But it's also important to be a little more pragmatic and know what *qualities* and *character* you are marrying. A marriage is supposed to last a lifetime; don't leave it to chance or to a competition over who can sweep you off your feet the best. If you don't know what you are looking for, you wouldn't know where to look.

At some point after my divorce was settled, my parents confessed they had known from the start that my marriage to John was a mistake. They could clearly see it from the sidelines but were afraid to talk to me about it. They felt responsible for not preventing my pain and were terribly sorry. To be honest, I am not sure I would have broken up with John even had my parents warned me of the potential outcome. I would have found a way to convince myself that we would see through whatever trials and tribulations we would encounter. After all, I believed we were in love and *what could go wrong when you are in love?* Boy, was I in for an expensive lesson.

THE PRICE OF SETTLING
NATALIE'S STORY

When it came to relationships, I settled and paid a hefty price. I was with Zack for ten years despite knowing deep down that he wasn't right for me. He treated me well, and I had already invested a whole decade of my prime years. I felt I was too old to go back to the dating scene and was afraid to start from scratch.

Where would I even meet new people? I was terrified of being single for the rest of my life.

He treated me well. That phrase kept me afloat.

And that's all there was. He treated *me* well, but he was rude to everyone else—my family *and* my friends. He saw no wrong with insulting my friends to their faces, making meals extremely uncomfortable. It got to a point where no one wanted to meet up with me anymore unless I came alone. My life became awkwardly divided. There was no safe place where Zack and my friends could civilly co-exist. He always found a way to offend someone with enough arrogance for the entire room. It was devasting for me to realize I was one of those gals whose friends and family despised their boyfriend. No one bothered to ask about him, and I learned it was best not to let his name come up. It was better to leave that part of my life unspoken. My friends had to gingerly dance around topics that may somehow relate to Zack; someone had to strategically but unnaturally change the subject.

I knew it hurt my friends and my family to see me that way. They felt I could do better and be so much happier. I knew they believed Zack didn't deserve me. They never explicitly expressed it, but I knew. And I was embarrassed that I wasn't truly happy because of my compartmental-ized life. Worse yet, I knew I was to blame for allowing it to be that way.

Still, I never left him because the fear of wasting time and being single forever overshadowed everything. Plus, I truly loved him. Others may not have understood why I could love such a person, but my feelings for him were real. I had believed Zack could change, and things would improve.

It never did.

I understood the problem wasn't so much that I had believed Zack could change. Rather, the problem was I believed he *wanted* to change. In reality, he never thought there was anything wrong with him. He never cared enough about the other valuable relationships in my life to try to be a part of them, or at a minimum, make peace. In hindsight, I had known this all along. I chose not to believe it'd have a lasting impact on my life, on my relationships with others, and my happiness. I had hung on to this false hope that it could be better one day. But that hope had no grounds; there were never any indications that things *would* get better. It was just an illusion I had permitted.

It was fortunate that we chose not to have children. I couldn't imagine having miniature versions of him. Either the kids would naturally learn to treat others as he did, or I would have had to continue to teach the kids not to be like him. Both seemed like terrible options.

If I could do it all over again, I would have convinced myself that being single forever is many times better than being unhappy forever. And that wasting ten years is noth-ing compared to wasting a lifetime.

MISMATCHED INTENTIONS
RON & LILY'S STORY

Ron and I were inseparable since day one. We dated for about eight years, then decided to move in together. I had always thought I would have been married by that age, but I didn't want to rush Ron into a marriage if we weren't ready. To be accurate, I was ready to get married and start a family, but it was obvious Ron wasn't. So, living together seemed like a good compromise.

Questions like "*when will they tie the knot?*" didn't ease up after we lived under one roof. If anything, it intensified. All the curious friends and nosy relatives pressed on to find out when the *big day* was. It became increasingly awkward because you can only say, "I don't know," in so many ways.

And I, in turn, asked Ron the same question. *When are we going to get married?*

Each time, he found new and creative ways to dodge the topic. It started to feel like I was begging someone to take me as his wife.

My eagerness had no mercy on me at all. I turned every little thing into a fantasy of how it would be the ultimate marriage proposal. When Ron had to run out to the store, I speculated that he would come back with a diamond ring. He came back with hair gel instead. It turned out the store was only the drug store.

When Ron asked me out on a dinner date, I was so sure this would be *the* night. I envisioned him on one knee, and I imagined how I would say yes, with just the right amount of surprise and enthusiasm. I had gotten teary-eyed just from *thinking* that I was finally going to be engaged. It turned

216

out Ron knew I had a stressful week at work and wanted to cheer me up. A beautiful gesture, but not beautiful enough.

And there was the time when Ron brought me breakfast in bed. It was a first. Of course, I immediately suspected something was up. I stealthily searched through every possible item on the tray, looking for the ring. *Nothing.* I even imagined it in the orange juice; some movies show the engagement ring in a glass of champagne. But the breakfast was only breakfast. Ron had found a new recipe he wanted to try, and of all days, I happened to sleep in that morning, so he brought it to me in bed.

No doubt, Ron was a sweet guy. However, he had no intention to marry me. After living together for five years, I finally had to be brutally honest with myself. There was no desire on his part to move forward, to start a family. He would rather evade the marriage questions than have an open conversation to tell me he simply had no plan to make me his wife. I couldn't shake the feeling he was waiting for something better to come along.

Sometimes, it takes a while to accept what's happening and decide to move on. For me, it took too long. I didn't know how, but I eventually gathered up the courage and walked out. And guess what? He didn't chase me back.

As I was still picking up pieces of my broken heart and mending my self-esteem, I unexpectedly met someone new. I warned him from the start that I wasn't ready and didn't want to date while on the rebound. He waited patiently for me, so sure we were meant to be.

Fast forward to three years later, and we were happily married. We had a lot in common, and our values aligned almost perfectly, especially our plan to have a loving home with four children. I adored his family, and he adored mine. For the first time in a long while, I felt *fully* appreciated and cherished. He had married me because he wanted to spend the rest of his life with me, *as his wife.*

My younger self suffered much longer than she should have with feelings of inadequacy. Looking back, I applauded her courage to make the difficult decision to break out of a dead-end relationship. I could not fault Ron for any of it and was grateful he had cared for me, but I saw we were clearly misaligned. We left important life choices undiscussed and made the wrong assumptions about each other. Ron had assumed I would be happy with the status quo for the rest of our lives; I had assumed he wanted a traditional family as much as I did.

You'll never find the right person if you never let go of the wrong one.

—Unknown

TAKEAWAYS

- Don't choose a spouse based only on feelings. Understand what qualities and values are important to you in a spouse.

- Seek input from people you respect and who care about your well-being.

- Do not settle. Marriage is for a lifetime. Do not make the decision lightly.

19

PARENTS ARE HUMAN TOO

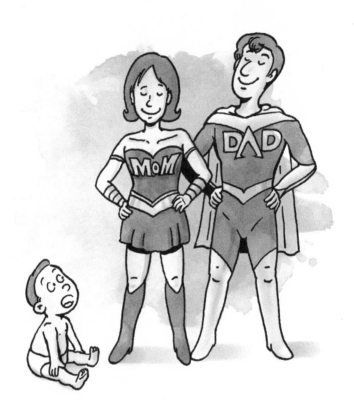

Parenting is the easiest thing in the world to have an opinion about, but the hardest thing in the world to do.

—Matt Walsh

We might think that our parents are often too hard on us or overly critical, but if we stop and think about it, we could very well be doing the same to them. Kids tend to think: *One day when I have kids, I will raise them differently.* It's as though we already have it figured out before we become parents ourselves. We have the common perception that our kids would turn out better as long as we do what our parents *didn't* do (or vice versa).

It seems more the exception than the norm to think that our parents know more than we do and that their life experiences actually mean something. Perhaps this is more prominent in the rebellious teenage years that parents look forward to *so* much when their sweet child transforms into an aloof stranger. And perhaps it's amplified by the expansion of technological development. The more technology advances, the more the older generation has a hard time keeping up. Imagine people who grew up with old rotary phones (look that up if you don't know what that is!) trying to adapt to using the latest smartphone with ease. As we become the ones who have to teach our parents these new technologies, we may see more role reversals—we are now the teacher and them the student.

Usually, parents are our biggest fans, advocators, and supporters. While this may not be the case for all parents, most parents want what's best for their children. We could save ourselves a lot of regrets by respecting and appreciating our parents' advice, wisdom, and knowledge while we are young.

ENDLESS SACRIFICES

Your parents have made countless sacrifices for you. It would be a mistake to think you deserve them or that it's only right they made those sacrifices because they were a *choice* your parents made. After having kids, I understand there are sacrifices every single day. Would I rather spend $200 and indulge in an awesome seafood feast, or would it be better to spend the money on ballet or soccer for my kids? Should I spend $15 for lunch, or is it wiser to set that money aside as investment for my daughter's college? How long do I keep wearing my scuffed, worn-out soled, embarrassing dress shoes before I replace them, instead of spending it on groceries? The *unspeakable* act of giving up my daily Starbucks™ lattes in exchange for free brewed coffee in the office freed up $30 a week, $120 a month, $1,440 a year to put toward my kids' school tuition.

When you stop *expecting* these sacrifices, you may find you appreciate them more. If there is only enough to spend on one new outfit, most mothers would rather let the daughter shine.

Yet somehow, we expect our parents to live perfect lives, set perfect examples, and cater to all our needs—when and how we want them. We frequently forget they, too, have emotions and feelings.

We expect grace from them but often give back little in return.

From the moment a newborn arrives, other things go on the backburner to focus on caring for the baby. As time goes on, kids remain the center of attention and are rarely denied anything. It soon becomes an expectation.

Unfortunately, it's not uncommon for this attitude to stick with us as we get older. Even as we become more independent, our expectations rarely decrease. In fact, as we enter our teenage years, we may continue to expect their unconditional love to include providing for our materialistic needs.

Kudos to parents who are able to provide to their kids to the fullest. I would like to encourage the children on the receiving end to take a moment to recognize how great their parents are for what they do, every single day. Have gratitude. Let's not wait until old age to realize the importance of giving them the credit they deserve.

It always amazes me to hear stories of immigrants arriving in a new country with hopes of a better life for their families and brighter futures for their children. So many leave the comforts of their homes and everything familiar to enter foreign land with $20 or $30 in their pockets. They force themselves to be resourceful and opportunistic to make ends meet, working until every part of their bodies ache. This incredible sacrifice summarizes the limitless power of a parent's love. They know that they have to make it work because of the dream to give their children a better life.

People often say that children grow up so fast. But our parents are growing older at the same pace. So many of us lead busy lives nowadays, but we cannot allow our schedules to be so busy it doesn't leave time for our parents. They need our unconditional love too. When they pass, I hope you will remember the loving, tender moments, and the lessons that will stick with you for life. Hold them close when you can, all the way to the very end. And know they loved you first, more than you'll ever know.

GRANDPARENTS ARE GEMS

Grandparents are gems. Their love is like an amplified version of a parent's love. They want to cuddle, snuggle, and spoil you, but their wisdom stems from generations of experience and learning. Not everyone has the opportunity to know their grandparents, or maybe distance separates them. By the time I was born, two of my grandparents had already passed away. Another was estranged, so that left me with only one grandparent—my maternal grandmother. I didn't live near my grandmother, so I didn't get to spend much time with her. But I recall some of the stories she told from when she was young. She tried not to dwell on the hardships she had endured, especially raising her family under extreme financial duress. There were times when I grew impatient when she went on and on with her life lessons. As a teenager, I didn't quite have the maturity to appreciate what she was doing—trying to instill wisdom within me that she had picked up along her journey. Now I understand that she, too, acknowledged that our days together were numbered, and she took every opportunity to share what she had learned in hopes of helping me get ahead, to be wiser. It was her way of giving me a glimpse into her past, my ancestry, to have a better view of the events that shaped our family. I learned how my past generations, despite a lack of education, overcame obstacles and built up noble characters through perseverance.

I lost my grandmother in my early twenties. It wasn't until then that I noticed how many of my peers still had their four grandparents alive and fully involved in their lives. I secretly wished they truly cherished their grandparents like rare gems.

OUR ROLES REVERSE AS OUR PARENTS AGE
ELISA'S STORY

During the death of my mother, I saw a mix of emotions in her eyes—sadness to say goodbye, relief to soon be rid of pain and suffering, worry for me and the rest of the family, gladness she would soon reunite with my dad. I also caught a glimpse of fear, perhaps of the unknown of what's next. In that instance, I realized I had become the source of strength. All my life, my mother had been the pillar, the glue in the family, the comforting voice who told me and my siblings everything would be all right. It was agonizing to see my mother drift away. There was something very final about this moment. It felt like there was suddenly a lot that I hadn't yet told her. The knowledge that I soon would not have a mother in my life shattered my heart. But this moment wasn't about me. I summoned all my strength to smile for my mother, squeezing her hand to give her the same reassurance she had always given us: "Everything will be all right."

THE POWER OF PARENTS' LOVE
AMANDA'S STORY

I had a strong relationship with my family until my teenage years when my friends became the most important people in my life. Being cool was a priority, and I started hanging out with the wrong crowd. I dated a lot of different guys who gave me attention and compliments. One thing led to another, and I ultimately became a teen mom at the tender age of sixteen. I will never forget the terror I felt when I realized I was pregnant. There was no turning back from that point. I didn't even want to imagine what my future would look like.

Not knowing what to do, I went to my friends for help, but they shamelessly abandoned me at the first sign of trouble. They had no interest in helping me out at a time when I needed the most support.

I eventually had to tell my parents the truth. It was the hardest thing I've ever had to do, looking them in the eye and confessing my big mistake. There were tears and disbelief and anger and *more* tears. For the first time, I saw my parents completely helpless. And I hated myself for putting them through this situation.

Suddenly, my mom stood up, walked toward me, and embraced me. She sobbed into my shoulder, and it was a weird realization just how much I had grown, and how long it had been since I last hugged my mom.

My mom didn't let go for a long, long time. I know she did it more for me rather than for herself. She knew I needed the hug, the reassurance that I was loved.

This happened about twenty years ago when society was not as accepting of teen pregnancies. My parents tolerated the dirty looks people freely gave at the sight of an under-aged mom and escorted me to all of my doctor appointments, making sure I never had to go alone. They let their love overpower the anger and disappointment created by this huge, irreversible mistake I made. They forgave me. And they were there through the even tougher times ahead— when the baby arrived and needed constant care. No one ever imagines this could happen to them; we certainly never did. But together as a family, we conquered one of the roughest patches of my life. And my appreciation for my parents was beyond measure.

Love your parents. We are so busy growing up, we often forget they are also growing old.

—Unknown

TAKEAWAYS

- Be gracious toward your parents. Allow them to be imperfect, just like we are imperfect.

- Appreciate all the sacrifices that your parents have made for you. Understand these were from choices they made, not just something you are entitled to.

- Make time for your parents and grandparents. They long to be loved too.

20

SAY I LOVE YOU OFTEN

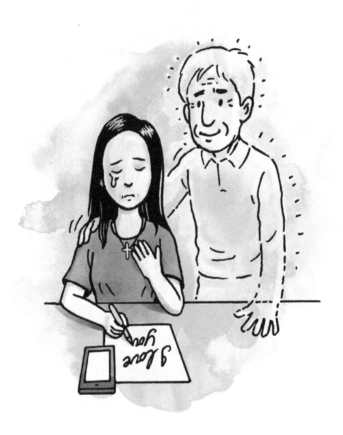

If there ever comes a day when we can't be together, keep me in your heart, I'll stay there forever.

—Winnie the Pooh by A. A. Milne

MY STORY

It was getting late in the day, and people started to make their way home from the office. I was waiting to escort a vendor team up to the boardroom to make their pitch. It was to be the start of a great partnership with an expert in the industry, enabling significant improvement for our company. I was nervous, though I wasn't the one making the presentation. This was my baby—I brought the idea to what it was that evening.

A message popped up on my phone telling me my dad, thousands of miles away, was in serious condition.

It was my uncle, suggesting—*urging*—I start considering coming back to see my dad.

The next message: "Here is a photo of your dad."

I was too afraid to open the image on my phone.

Staying focused during the presentation was a struggle. I tried hard not to imagine what the photo of my dad looked like.

The presentation was a success, and we got approval to move ahead with the project. This was a monumental moment, especially for my career, but all I could think about was my dad.

My sister on the other side of the world had received a similar update from my uncle. She and I began to converse on synchronizing our flights to head home.

Within a few hours, we got the news that most children dread. Our dad had suddenly passed away.

Our search for flights home became more urgent, interrupted by pure shock as we tried to make sense of what happened. Every few minutes or so, I gave in, curled up, and wept.

They say it's possible to cry so much you run out of tears. That was certainly not the case that night.

The flight home was awful. So many times I broke down and sobbed. I was in a daze, still trying to come to terms with my new reality. I was so grateful my husband was there with me the entire time. His silent embrace reminded me I wasn't going through this alone. He didn't try to convince me that everything was okay because we both knew it wasn't. Instead, he cried with me.

A few months prior, my dad had been receiving therapy for his cancer and was wrapping up his last session. He was so close to completing his treatments so he could move on to focusing his time and energy on his recovery. The treatments often left him breathless, completely exhausted, and almost lifeless as he laid curled up in a fetal position, wishing the pain and discomfort would go away. He wished for life to be normal again.

His cancer was only stage 1 at diagnosis. On a scale of 0 to 4, stage 1 should imply a very good chance of survival.

And that was what my dad had—a great chance at being healthy again. But the chemotherapy compromised his immunity so much that when he contracted a severe bacterial infection, his body had no strength left to fight it, and he ultimately lost his life.

I still recall the last time I spent with my dad. It was during an especially long visit to be there for him as he underwent the longest stretch of his treatments. My boss at the time, being as awesome and empathetic as he had always been, made special arrangements for me to work remotely during this time. I was able to sit alongside my dad as he received his daily injection as part of his chemotherapy. He tried his best to make it seem like there was nothing to it as the medical staff injected a needle into a vein on the back of his hand. But I could tell it was hitting his body hard. His vein closed by the third day, and they had to try a new vein; his jaw tightened, trying to hide his anxiety as he sucked on ice chips. He didn't want his daughter to see him in such a vulnerable state. But I am thankful I could be there to hold his free hand—as the other one slowly transported chemicals through his body, killing the cancerous cells along with the good ones. I honestly could not remember the last time I held my dad's hand. It could have been when I was a little girl.

Another time, we were sitting together in the hospital waiting area, listening for his name for his radiotherapy appointment. Out of the blue, he pondered out loud when it would be time for him and my mom to sell the house I grew up in and downsize to a condo.

"It might be more comfortable to live my remaining twenty years in a condo rather than a house."

He must have noticed the wave of sadness that washed over me because he continued, "Well, if we are honest, living another twenty years would already be quite good, don't you think? That would bring me to my mid-eighties, and that's truly already a good life."

We sat in silence for a few seconds, deep in our thoughts. I can only imagine what was going through his mind—perhaps what the next twenty years would entail. I wonder if he thought about how his life would ultimately end and whether he would be scared when the time came. I was still trying to process the concept of losing a parent.

He did not have another twenty years and passed away just over a month later. And he was two months away from retiring. *Two months*. My parents worked so hard all their lives to make ends meet and hardly had a chance to enjoy life or travel. Their dream was to start traveling after retirement. And they were so close to living that dream.

Sadly, while alone, my mom had to go through the trauma of hearing her husband only had hours to live. She stayed by my dad's side as he was in the hospital. What a blessing she could be there with him and be that loving wife my dad so very much needed. They continued to laugh and share jokes until my dad lost consciousness. And there was no better way to manifest their marriage vows: "till death do us part."

There were family and a few close friends with my mom in the hospital during the final moments with my dad, and for that, I am eternally grateful she didn't have to go through that alone. She had shoulders to cry on, embraces to lean into.

The days that followed were a blur. We kept busy toggling between preparing for the funeral (who knew there was so much involved?), notifying friends and family, and starting the process of putting away my dad's things. There wasn't much quiet time to absorb reality and deal with our grief. It's not easy losing a parent, especially when the death is sudden and unexpected, and you didn't have a chance to say goodbye. I'm not sure there really is a way to prepare for the pain of losing a parent, a pillar in your life, someone who's been there for you since you were born.

My dad was well-loved. It was largely because he had a way of making people feel at ease, loved, and appreciated. He was the kind of guy who picked up items left on the floor at the grocery store and would fix things for you without calling attention to it. One time, my parents stayed over at a friend's house while visiting their hometown. By the time they left, the door magically stopped squeaking, kitchen cabinet hinges had tightened, cabinet doors had straightened, and the bathroom faucet stopped leaking. This good friend of my dad's, who had known him for decades, instantly recognized the hands behind the work. It was a work full of love that didn't need acknowledgment.

During my last visit, my dad still took the time to wash grapes, cut up apples, and deliver them to my workspace. From the sound of slow, heavy footsteps up the stairs, I could tell he should have been lying down to rest. Instead, he chose to burn some of his limited energy to do what he could to care for me, to help nourish my body. He put my health above his.

The night before I left, my dad sadly told me that he wouldn't be able to take me to the airport in the morning.

There was a silent understanding his body was simply too exhausted to even sit in the car for an extended ride. That's how much the effects of his treatments wore down his body. I hugged him and felt the frailness of his thinning body. It was as though I had to hold back from squeezing him too hard in case it would hurt him. My dad was a strong, brave fighter. But the evidence of this tiring battle was too much to hide. I jokingly told him, "Be good now!" He smiled and said, "I will." We didn't verbally express our love because it wasn't something we did as a family except inside greeting cards and correspondence. How I wish I had told my dad that I loved him. I wish I had told him how grateful I was to have him as my father and for the unconditional love and support he had given me my whole life. Now I go by the faith that he simply knew. And gosh, how I wish I could tell him just how much I miss him, his gentle smile.

Hearing "your dad died" was not something I had anticipated hearing in my thirties. I didn't even have my first child yet. As each year goes by, I cherish our photos more and more from my wedding, dancing our father-daughter dance. There was indescribable joy in our eyes. One photograph specifically caught me glancing upward toward the sky, my expression full of gratefulness for my Heavenly Father as I embraced my earthly father.

I lamented that my children would not have the opportunity to get to know my dad, to see his kindness and gentleness with their own eyes, to witness the ways he served others voluntarily and often surreptitiously. My best friend, full of wisdom as she always has been, reminded me it was up to me to live out his legacy, that my kids would get to know my dad through me, my actions, and the stories I share. They would have the opportunity to see my dad's acts of kindness through my hands and my generosity. They would get to understand their grandpa's love through my love.

The death of any loved parent is an incalculable lasting blow. Because no one ever loves you again like that.

—Brenda Ueland

TAKEAWAYS

- Take every opportunity to tell people you care about that you love them.

- We cannot anticipate when someone may no longer be around. Appreciate them while you can.

- Cherish your parents and grandparents. They love you like no one else does.

21

EACH AGE LASTS ONLY ONE YEAR

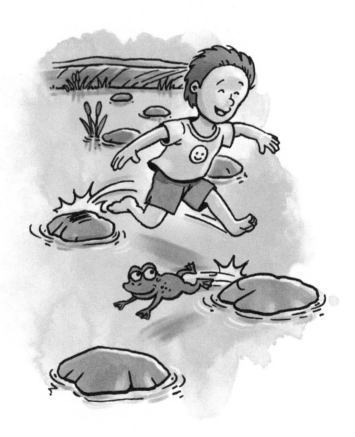

Time waits for no one.

—Yasutaka Tsutsui

Looking back at our younger years, how many of us rushed time to move along quickly so we could grow up faster? Isn't this one of life's greatest ironies? When we are young, we yearn to be older. Yet when we are old, we ache for the possibility to be young again.

We have exactly one year to enjoy each age. Every four years, we get a bonus day for leap year. But that's it—just one year. No more, no less. And by thinking about it in that manner, perhaps we may appreciate each day, each month, each season a little more. There will not be another *summer when I was eight years old,* or *the winter when I was eighteen, my baby's first year as an infant,* or *the spring break when my son was ten,* or *the party when we celebrated my mom's seventy-fifth birthday.* All these milestones pass as quickly as they come. And once they pass, they are gone forever. Memories are all that is left.

Nor will there be a repeat of firsts. Your first of anything will be just that—a first. Embrace the excitement in these firsts, even if they may be daunting. You choose whether to welcome them with dread or enthusiasm, to face them with a let's-get-it-over-with attitude, or view them as the beginning of a new chapter despite the unknowns.

I recently read an article about your lasts. Now, that's not something we think about often. It spoke of things we don't realize are our last until they're gone—the last time we see certain friends, the last time we set foot in a school, the last time you talk to a friend, the last time we carry our child, the last time we hear someone's voice, or the last time we embrace a loved one.

So, cherish every year. Regardless of what age you are now, vow to cherish your tomorrow, your next week, and your next month more than you ever have before. Each new day we wake up to is, in fact, *a gift*, so treat it as such. A gift is not guaranteed, and we should appreciate each one.

Don't rush to grow up. You'll get there soon enough. One year isn't much time. It's fifty-two weeks. If Saturday is your favorite day, there are only fifty-two of those to enjoy each year. If you live to eighty, you will have only enjoyed, at most, eighty springs, eighty summers, eighty autumns, and eighty winters by the time you leave earth. Some of those, if not most, may simply be fleeting memories. So while you can, make the most of it.

REGRETS

It seems the older we get, the more regrets we have. Perhaps simply living more days offer more opportunities for us to look back and wish things were different, that we had done something or hadn't done something. For some of these regrets, it could be because of a particular event or decision that ultimately changed the rest of our lives forever. For others, it boils down to how we spent our time.

When we are young, we tend to consider time as an infinite resource. There is less of an urgency to get things done, especially when there is no assigned deadline. Self-discipline is still a work-in-progress virtue. But as we get older, we start to see time as not quite so limitless after all. We can no longer live like a child, with a wake-up-and-play-and-eat-and-play-again-and-eat-some-more-and-go-to-sleep-and-repeat kind of lifestyle. As we reach more milestones in life, we may encounter moments where it is too late to accomplish certain things. There are things we cannot redo—we cannot relive a certain age or redo a lot of our firsts. We cannot go back in time to correct bad choices.

If we can be more intentional with the way we use our time, it may help us avoid some regrets. Planning can help greatly. Plan your days, months, and years with purpose. Be in the driver's seat about how to spend your life and decide in advance. Sure, sometimes our plans go awry, but if you have your path more-or-less set out, it's easier to get back on track if you find yourself starting to veer off. This can help eliminate meaningless, time-consuming things.

TIME IS AN ASSET

Time is the one thing we can't *ever* get back. Once it's gone, it's gone. Time is finite within each of our lifespans. There is no way to produce more.

A lot of people talk about time management, but we cannot truly manage time. Time moves on regardless of what we choose to do with it. We are just along for the ride. It's our *attention* that we can manage.

When I was young, I thought time was infinite. So, one summer in high school, I spent the majority of my time watching TV, binging on junk food, and lazing around. Sure, I did some reading here and there, but my friends were earning extra credits to accelerate their education. I could have followed their path and graduated earlier, too, but at the time I didn't feel the urgency. Now, married with two kids and a fulltime job, I cringe to think that at that age, I felt I *deserved* an extensive break. Boy, do I wish I could take a break now.

Time seems to go faster as we get older. Perhaps this is due to an increase in responsibilities and tasks, the exponential growth in consumable information, the rapid advancement of technology causing everything to move so much more rapidly, or perhaps a combination of all the above. Regardless, it seems increasingly challenging to pause and appreciate life. Time management seems more of an elusive concept than something truly attainable. The list of to-dos grows faster than we can complete them.

A lot of times, it comes to prioritization. Prioritize your long list of tasks, evaluate the lower ranking ones, and determine whether you can defer or eliminate those. We tend to allocate time to certain tasks because it's on our list and not because they're truly important. Streamline where possible. Sometimes *good enough* is okay!

Time is the most precious gift you can give. It's more significant than things money can buy because you can replenish money, but you cannot replenish time. So, go and spend time *with* people and *on* people. Show them you care and they matter because you are giving them *time*, your most valuable resource.

By no means do I mean to imply that life is smooth sailing all the time. There will be peaks and valleys. Some seasons can be hard to enjoy, and we want them to go by quickly. Other days seem to slow to a crawl like we are on an uphill climb with no light at the end of the tunnel. A friend of mine once told me about her sister who suffered from a muscular disorder. Physical movements alone caused a lot of pain. Instead of choosing to lie in bed and mope her life away, she chose to get up early every day and spent at least eight hours a day reaching out to people in need and prayed for them. She felt that if she couldn't physically help and support people, she could help sustain people spiritually through prayer. Despite her mobility limitations, she chose not to allow those to prevent her from spending her time well, maximizing each day to help others. That was her way of living her life to the fullest.

I hope this inspires you. Don't underestimate the ripple effect of how you choose to spend your time. Your actions could very well inspire others, which, in turn, could further inspire even more. Wouldn't it be beautiful if there is no end to this relay in life?

Don't rush through life. Time is a gift. Remember, you have all but one year to enjoy each age. Make the most of it.

WHEN KIDS COME EARLY
OLIVIA AND PATRICK'S STORY

We were high school sweethearts and dated through college. Through that time, we saw the way our friends navigated through the dating scene, met new people, and went through bad breakups. It served us well because it made us very grateful for having known early on that we wanted to marry each other.

We got married when we were twenty-two. There was a bit of a *why wait?* mentality. Both sets of parents were supportive, particularly as we were fresh out of college graduations and so young.

We planned to work for at least five years, get our career off to a solid start, then begin building our family. By then, we anticipated that we would be in a better financial stage to cover all the expenses that come with a child. We worked toward having Olivia switch to part-time so she could spend more time with our baby. And we had agreed on having two children, so that would mean we become parents when we are twenty-eight and have our second and final child at thirty. It seemed reasonable to us. It may even allow us to travel once or twice before we buckled down.

Well, that didn't quite go according to plan. We soon found ourselves pregnant while at our entry-level jobs. Our finances didn't allow us to afford childcare. We felt like kids who had to grow up overnight, from relying on our parents to now having a little person be completely dependent on us for survival. It was overwhelming, to say the least. Our little studio apartment was too small, but we stuck with it for as long as we could; it was a good thing an infant didn't take up much space.

To stick with the plan of having our children two years apart, we had our second child two years after, when we were twenty-five. And then, we were done when a lot of our friends were still floundering, some searching for their future spouse, others not wanting to settle down for another ten years. They were living their best life with no strings attached, starting to have money to party and travel to their heart's desire.

We felt a little out of place hanging out with the same crowd. While others talked about the latest restaurant and clubs, we were barely surviving through the intense sleep deprivation, baby burp-ups, and endless dirty diapers. Eating out also became a luxury; we had so many more expenses as parents. When our friends talked about their latest travels, we could only nod—slightly in envy—and imagined seeing these places for ourselves. Undoubtedly, it became harder to relate to the rest of our friends.

Having a child at twenty-three years old meant we were parents to a teenager while in our thirties. I attribute the closeness of our relationship to the closeness of our age. It's easier to relate to a teen when in your thirties. A lot of people commented we looked like siblings, and it was true. We hung out and talked like friends, but our children maintained an underlying reverence for us, something we worked hard to protect. Of course, there were ugly days, but for the most part, it was wonderful raising them as young parents.

When our kids were in college, some of our friends had only recently gotten married, and some were starting or trying to start a family. True, we fumbled a lot as young parents when trying to figure it out. Most days we really didn't know what we were doing. We were immature beings trying to grow up ourselves! We hadn't gone out to see the world and hadn't spent much on ourselves, so everything in our house was pretty much bare bones. Again and again, we failed but kept trying because giving up wasn't exactly an option. With the help of friends and family, along with a solid marriage that allowed a great partnership, we made it through. And judging from the relationship we have been able to sustain with our now-adult children, we'd argue we made it through with flying colors.

Some of our friends believed we had wasted away our youth, robbing ourselves of the experiences, resources, and freedom we *could have* spent on ourselves during prime years. They thought we were foolish to tie ourselves down so early, give up everything, and invest it all in our children instead. There were times when we did feel like we were missing out, that we didn't know what it was like to be in your twenties and be *out there having fun* without a care in the world. But then, we'd pause, take a good look at our children, and honestly conclude that we really wouldn't have traded this life for anything else.

There is a good chance we will still be fairly young when we become grandparents. And God willing, we might even live to become great-grandparents! What a blessing it could be to see not only the next generation but the one after that, *and the one after that.* It would make all the struggles as young parents completely worthwhile.

DON'T WAIT FOR ENOUGH
HANNAH AND JIM'S STORY

We dated a lot before finally meeting each other. We were in our late thirties by the time we got married. Hannah had always known she wanted to marry early, ideally before thirty, but all the serial dating never yielded someone worth marrying. Jim, on the other hand, wanted to date for as long as possible, but by the time he turned thirty-nine, his mindset changed. It was like his biological clock went off. He wanted to settle down but hadn't found anyone he would have wanted to marry and wished he had taken dating more seriously. That time could have been put to better use to evaluate the kind of wife he wanted instead of going out with *just anyone* who seemed fun.

Because we got married rather late in life, we soon found ourselves struggling to conceive. Our doctor advised us not to wait too long before considering fertility help unless we wanted to consider adopting instead. It was devastating; we had never imagined we might not be able to have biological children because we're *too old*. Weren't we still part of the dating scene not too long ago?

We ultimately decided to receive fertility assistance. Hannah became pregnant at forty-one and gave birth when she was forty-two years old. It might not sound too old given how common it is for older women to have children today, but the energy level at forty-two is nothing compared to how it was in the twenties or thirties. And kids demand *a lot* of energy.

Looking ahead, we will be in our sixties when our daughter graduates from college. We may look like their friends' grandparents and may actually be their age!

It wasn't exactly our choice that we didn't meet each other until so late in our lives, and we would not hesitate to say that our marriage was worth the wait. But some people wait on purpose, thinking they need to make more money, travel, or enjoy life first. But there isn't *enough* money that will suddenly make you ready to have kids. It did help that we were both more established in our careers by the time we were married and could afford a bigger house with more space for a family, a cushier income than what we were making in our twenties, and we could give our children more options. And we were both quite well-traveled by the time we got married, which helps from a cultural sense. We had our fair share of fun as singles, so in a way, it's like we got it *out* of our system.

We saw some friends who started having kids earlier in life and finished paying college tuitions before turning fifty. Their *fun* and traveling started a little later than we did, but they got to do it with their children, who were at an age to appreciate the adventures.

Don't view having children as a buzzkill. Life can be so much more colorful with children; they truly bring indescribable joy. But they do require a lot of time and energy, both of which you have less of as you age. So many days we wanted to sit back and watch our daughter play because our energy couldn't keep up, no matter how caffeinated we were. But what our daughter needed were involved parents, not couch parents. Perhaps if we were younger, we could have given our daughter a sibling or two, so they'd have companions for life.

Grant your children the gift of having more years with you. Allow your grandchildren the privilege of being able to know you in person and not only through photographs and stories told by others.

WHAT'S THE BIG RUSH?
NANCY'S STORY

My husband and I raised four children who were fairly close in age. That meant every day had its craziness and challenges. All our children turned out to be great, caring individuals. But as I now spend time with my grandchildren, I realize how much I missed out on my children's childhoods because my mind was often not present. I spent a lot of energy trying to prepare for the next day and the following week. It was as though I was constantly combating chaos and tried to get ahead of it. This means I operated primarily in an auto-pilot mode and was not truly in the moment with my kids.

Life was one big rush. In our household, we often hollered, "*Hurry up!*" as though it was our battle cry.

As a grandmother now, the reality is I don't have the pressures of working a full-time job and trying to manage the household while raising the kids, paying bills, packing lunches and snacks, tending to school assignments, chauffeuring kids between school and extracurricular activities, plus what seems like a million more things. There is now less for me to do in general, so it makes sense that it's easier to sit and play with my grandchildren without my mind wandering to the next thing on my task list. However, it's within our control whether we are absentminded or not. When I was a busy mother of four, I may not have had the luxury to spend three hours every night playing with my children, but I know I could have done better to be 100% focused on them during our interactions.

To my younger self, I wish I could tell you moments with your kids are limited and pass by so quickly. I know you know this already but allow me to reiterate. Please understand the gravity of my words. It's true when they say that the days are long, but the years are short. They really are! As you hold your newborn in your arms, enduring those long nights when all she did was cry, know that those will soon pass as well. Some days will feel endless, like you are digging from a well that has already run dry. But it won't be too far into the future when you will think back and miss those moments when you did nothing else but hold and rock your baby. She won't remember those tender moments—they are for you to hang on to. Pay attention to that sweet baby scent and try to engrain it into your memory. There will come a day when you can barely recall the lovely fragrance of your newborn or the feel of this small, vulnerable life wrapped up in your arms, her heartbeat responding to yours.

Don't waste time on the things that don't carry meaning. Sure, some chores don't go away (and never will), but perhaps we can perceive those as an opportunity to take mental breaks or as teaching moments for your children. Focus the time you have to be intentional about making lasting memories and building a strong relationship with your children. When they request your undivided attention, stop what you're doing and tune in. Be the mother they need you to be, right then and there. You might not be able to give them everything they want, and that's okay! But try to carve out time for your children, find ways to include them as you run errands, take each chance in your everyday life to teach them and talk to them, and make the most of the days you have with them. Those days are numbered. And your children are certainly worth your time.

> *Time is free, but it's priceless. You can't own it, but you can use it. You can't keep it, but you can spend it. Once you've lost it, you can never get it back.*
>
> —Harvey Mackay

TAKEAWAYS

- You have 365 days to enjoy each age. Make the most of it. There are no re-dos.

- Invest spending time with your loved ones. Those moments are fleeting. Make memories while you can.

- Time is precious. It is the best gift you can give.

22

YOU ARE WONDERFULLY MADE

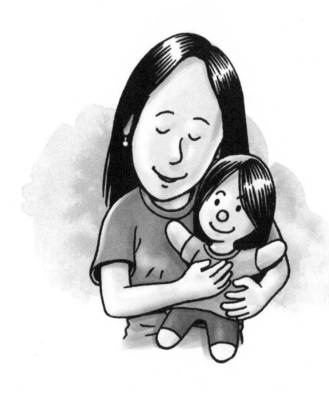

Dear Younger Me,

I want you to know how proud I am of you and how far you've come.

Please also know you are wonderfully made. You are unique *by design*. Of all the lessons within this book, this is the most important.

You were created for a purpose. It is your responsibility to navigate through your life to find that purpose. Reflect on your path often and be honest about whether it takes you to where you need to go. Sometimes changing course can be challenging, perhaps even painful, but you have the courage and strength deep inside to do just that. So, if you notice you're going off course, be bold and intentional, reset your path, and make good, wise choices for the sake of your future. Recognize the power of consequences, good or bad. Some can have a lasting impact on the rest of your life.

When you have setbacks, use those experiences to learn, not to give yourself an excuse to wallow in self-pity. Keep in mind that you have a great support system. We are created to be a part of a greater whole. So reach out! There are so many people willing to extend a hand, offer a hug, give you advice. But you need to reach out. Acknowledge when you need help, and don't let shame hold you back. Don't let *you* hold you back. I know you would generously help a friend without hesitation. And trust me when I say there are many out there who would do the same for you.

Nothing is impossible, even if it may feel that way. If it's important and if it's good, find a way to make it happen. Sometimes, it starts with sheer will. Lean on this book—and this chapter in particular—as a friend and guide. Read and apply the lessons and hold them close to your heart. There are many nuggets of wisdoms packed in these pages from a wide range of people who understand what you are going through and what you are about to go through. Now that you are armed with these *keys to creating a life you love*, what are you going to do with them?

Be gracious to others. And don't forget to be gracious to yourself.

On days when you feel like you are running on empty, alone, and struggling to push forward, know that I'm on the sidelines, cheering you on. *You are not alone!* You are valued. You are loved. *You are wonderfully made.* Your Creator watches over you, wanting so much for you to comprehend His love. His love for you is perfect. There is no other love like His. He pieced you together in the most perfect way, and you are worthy and magnificent.

Love,
Future You

ACKNOWLEDGMENTS

When I first felt the undeniable calling to publish this book, I took on this enormous project without truly understanding how much time and effort it would take. I have heard that a lot of people desire to write a book, but the majority of them never get there. I would have joined that statistic if not for the tremendous help and encouragement I received throughout the entire process.

First and foremost, I would like to thank my Heavenly Father for loving me despite my imperfections and for trusting me with this book.

I would also like to thank everyone who contributed to the book by providing their life lessons and stories, sharing wholeheartedly what they would tell their younger selves if they had a chance. Thank you for your transparency and generosity. The book is only possible with your input, especially those who not only provided their own stories but invited others in their network to do so. Thank you for your desire and enthusiasm to help the younger generation together.

To you, my reader, thank you for allowing me to be a part of your journey. I hope this book helps you, encourages you, and gives you hope. Always remember: *your future is in your hands*. Take it seriously, make wise choices, and ensure your future is in *good* hands.

Thank you to Author Academy Elite, for guiding me throughout the entire writing and publication process from when I first made the decision to publish a book but had zero knowledge on how to even get started, to having a book in hand with my name confidently printed on its cover. Thank you for helping to turn me from a dreamer to an official published author.

To my sounding boards, beta readers, and cheerleaders—Ai-Lin Ku, Ngoc Nguyen, Myra Pacubas, and Steve Schoen. I am thankful for your wisdom, honesty, and assistance. My sanity was saved because of you.

Special shout out goes out to my amazing editor, Felicity Fox, for your expertise and patience. Thank you for not only enabling my manuscript to be something I can be proud of (and cutting out thousands of unnecessary words that were mere noise) but also answering my millions of questions and giving me frequent doses of encouragement.

Thank you to my illustrator, Pottery Chan, for the brilliant artwork that brought this book to life. You understood my vision when I failed to express it through words and offered suggestions I never would have thought of. God knew I needed you on my team before I knew it myself.

I would like to thank Vivian Woo, my best friend of a hundred years (we're not that old but it sure feels like that's how long we have known each other). As I worked on this book, I was able to reflect what a positive influence you had on my life. Thank you for being my rock and source of wisdom all these years, keeping me grounded in what matters.

I would like to thank my parents from whom I have learned so, so much. You may not have had the opportunity to receive extensive education, but you taught through your own lives as role models. You instilled in me and my sister the virtues of hard work, integrity, and that it's better to give than to receive. You made our hearts full.

Thank you to my sister, Fatima Tsang, for always being the fearless one. You show me nothing is impossible when you put your mind to it. You've inspired me since we were young to go outside of my comfort zone. We may be geographically far apart, but I am forever grateful you are my sister.

To Christa and Jesse, it is truly a blessing to have the opportunity to be your mommy. You teach me so much in each of your fun, loving ways. Thank you for showing me grace and the power of quick forgiveness. I am excited to see what your futures hold . . . you are going to shine bright! Thank you for being so understanding every time Mommy had to "spend time on the book."

And to my love, Kevin, thank you for your support with this book. Squeezing the time out to dedicate to this book despite our crazy schedules meant a lot of sacrifices. I am grateful you stood with me to see this project through, choosing to believe with me there is a greater purpose to get it published. Thank you for being the creative one, proactively offering different perspectives and ideas I wouldn't have come up with. Thank you for the encouragement you have showered me along the way, for believing in me as an author, and for showing me it's important to turn something you are passionate about into something you do.

Made in the USA
Monee, IL
28 November 2021